The Shade Upon My Right Hand

THE SHADE UPON MY RIGHT HAND

by

Elizabeth Aijian Munroe

VANTAGE PRESS
New York / Washington / Atlanta
Los Angeles / Chicago

Biblical quotations are from the King James version of the Bible.

FIRST EDITION

Published by Vantage Press, Inc.
516 West 34th Street, New York, New York 10001

Manufactured in the United States of America
ISBN: 533-05359-5

Library of Congress Catalog Card No.: 82-90231

To the memory of my beloved parents, Siroon and Kaloost Aijian, from whom I caught the Christian faith, and to my wonderful husband, Tom, whose loving care has always seen me through. With special thanks to Pris, Jack, Chip, Karen, and Laurie, my best friends!

FOREWORD

This is a timely book, in that it fills a great need. Forty years of pastoral ministry convinces me of this; moreover, it is exceptionally readable.

There are some 240 million people in these United States, of whom some 52 percent are women. The percentage of women in nearly all church congregations is significantly larger. Of these some 130 million women, by present statistics, 11 percent will someday have a mastectomy. This is an enormous number. Also concerned are many times that number of husbands, families, and close friends. This is the potential audience for this book.

From a patient's point of view, there are few books in this field, and some of those few are decidedly not upbeat. This book is. It is the story of how a potentially devastating experience was turned into a life-enriching one by faith and hope and love and prayer.

This is achieved, not by any facile evading of the malignant and often fatal nature of the enemy, but by looking grim reality full in the face. Modern medicine and surgery are received gratefully as indispensable allies in the battle for her survival. They are acknowledged as God's partners and instruments in our healing . . . a sort of twentieth-century fulfillment of Jesus' promise that "the things you see me do, you shall do, and greater than these shall you do."

A word of introduction about the author: She and her family became members of our congregation and close friends during the last twenty years of my twenty-six-year pastorate. It is literally no exaggeration to say that she became, spiritually, one of the more beautiful people in that congregation. She is so generous in thought and deed, so charitable in her judgments, so genuine in her faith, so innocent in her joys, so warm in her appreciations, that she hardly seems real.

But she is real! There is a dark line like the shadow of a cross in her life. She is of Armenian stock. Her grandparents were martyred for their faith in the Turkish massacres before World War I. Her parents fled to America to save their lives. By their diligence, they prospered.

She met Tom Munroe at Trinity University, in San Antonio He "rushed" her in a fairytale romance. Being married to a character of such extravagant energy and sense of humor can help the saints remember their earthly roots. But their marriage is warm and supportive, a partnership in all things; they remain best friends even when the campgrounds turn to mud. From this story you will learn how supportive a husband—and family—can be at such times.

Liz is real! And her book is real! A talented artist and silversmith, she had no aspiration to write—and didn't know she could. But she writes of a searing experience in a fluid prose. The experience is so vivid it seems to have given her almost total recall. Her intuition has guided her into sharing those that are most helpful to others.

In Liz, there is no guile. She puts it all down without embarrassment—bedpans, vomiting, pain, the dazzling lights of the operating room, the jarring orange of her tasteless and ill-planned room, the psychological shock and long reluctance to face her own disfigurement.

Her generous spirit is reflected throughout. She finds less of the dismal hospital service, the revolting food, and surly personnel so much complained about. To her, the doctors are concerned, the nurses are efficient, the bathrooms are clean. Everywhere, she meets compassion and kindness. They are there to be helpful, and they are. Others, of course, have a different report of that same experience. I cannot help but conclude that Liz Munroe got what she gave and received what she expected: ". . . With what measure you mete out, it shall be measured unto you."

If you or a loved one or friend is facing such an experience, this is the best guide I know into the shadowed valley. These pages will prepare you to find, even there, green pastures and healing waters. I should add one note of preachment—if you would turn any of life's cruel tragedies into something of a triumph, be sure you have cultivated your faith and plowed your Bible as Liz has.

John D. Craig, Pastor Emeritus
Central Presbyterian Church
Houston, Texas

PREFACE

In the New Testament, the fourth chapter of the book of Acts, when the apostles Peter and John were commanded not to speak or teach in the name of Jesus Christ, their response was, ". . . we cannot but speak the things which we have seen and heard." I am able to identify with that kind of commitment and courage, having listened since early childhood to stories of grandparents and other family martyred for their Christian faith. My own faith has not been so tested; even so, I am compelled to speak. At no risk to myself, but rather at the insistence of the "still, small voice," I am compelled to speak of my own experience of mastectomy surgery, and of the faith that, once again, sustained me in perfect peace.

One out of every thirteen women faces mastectomy at some point in her lifetime. The prospect is unpleasant, and the surgery can be devastating. I have just joined the thousands of women who have undergone that surgery, and I have a statement to make about it. I "cannot but speak."

Surely some will ask who E. Munroe might be, or who she is to feel she is to write a book. I ask myself that same question! This book is a witness to my faith as a Christian, and how that faith has applied to one of life's desperate conditions. In my lifetime, I have known great sorrow, heartbreaking tragedy, and times of personal debility; through every difficult circumstance of life, I have also known the strength and peace that are ours in the Lord. There for all to claim, I want to speak of the joy of claiming, as I have found it to be so in my own experience.

Mine is a simple faith, for I have no background in theology and cannot consider myself an articulate person. My only wish is to share my story with others who face mastectomies, hopeful that I might encourage and comfort those who are in need. Perhaps my experience will hearten and support some in time of trouble. While none is excused from fear and doubt, sadness and pain, all may share in the great sustaining power of the Rock of our salvation; all may share in the promise of Christ that, if we are open, we shall surely receive:

> "Ask, and it shall be given you; seek, and ye shall find; knock, and it shall be opened unto you: For everyone that asketh receiveth; and he that seeketh findeth; and to him that knocketh it shall be opened." (Matthew 7:7, 8)

What a promise! It has been my comfort, hope, and refuge in every time of need, and I pray that it will be so for all who are seeking.

Elizabeth Aijian Munroe

CHAPTER ONE

"FOR WE ARE SAVED BY HOPE: BUT HOPE THAT IS SEEN IS NOT HOPE: FOR WHAT A MAN SEETH, WHY DOTH HE YET HOPE FOR?

BUT IF WE HOPE FOR THAT WE SEE NOT, THEN DO WE WITH PATIENCE WAIT FOR IT.

LIKEWISE, THE SPIRIT ALSO HELPETH OUR INFIRMITIES:

AND WE KNOW THAT ALL THINGS WORK TOGETHER FOR GOOD TO THEM THAT LOVE GOD, TO THEM WHO ARE CALLED ACCORDING TO HIS PURPOSE."

Romans 8:24–26b, 28

Yesterday the sword was removed from my side. I had expected to feel so well that I would want to begin on my book as soon as I returned home from the doctor's office. Instead, I was quite ill, running high fever and feeling more pain than I had experienced in the ten days since my surgery. "The sword" was the term I used to describe the pain caused by the drainage tubes that remained in my left side following my mastectomy, remaining longer than usual because the drainage had not yet stopped its flow into the hemo-vac. Dr. L. had assured me that I would be far more comfortable with the tubes left in my side a few days longer than I would be if he had to aspirate by needle the fluids that would accumulate there. I agreed emphatically.

The stress in the tissues surrounding the tubes was enough to cause the fever and pain, but now, hoping to lessen that stress, Dr. L. had told me to stop exercising my arm. I had been very conscientious about using my affected arm, because the nurses, as well as Dr. L., had emphasized the importance of the exercises to the arm. In the operating room, my arm had been tightly bound with elastic bandage as a precaution against swelling, but I still was faithful in trying to climb the walls with my fingers. So, because I had not used my arm for over twenty-four hours, it was more swollen and painful than it had been. I hugged it to my chest as Tom and I drove home in the gray dusk of Houston, creeping along in what is known as the five-o'clock traffic.

"I'm sorry that the removing of the tubes was so painful for you," he said with the compassion he had expressed all during our ordeal. He said that he had heard my cries from the doctor's office where he sat and was tempted to rush in and offer me protection.

"Well, I'm sorry that I wasn't able to contain the tears any better."

I had told Dr. L. that I was on the verge of tears when he began to remove my bandages, and that I was already worn out from the pain. When he pulled the tubes and they were released from my flesh, I howled with agony, sobbing as I had not done since my surgery.

Now that it was over, I told Tom that it reminded me of the Western movies in which the cowboy is mortally wounded with the arrow in his chest, and his buddy is called upon to yank it from his flesh. Both are very brave, of course. I wasn't.

"But," I complained," I didn't even have a bullet to bite on." We chuckled together as we inched our way closer to home.

Tom and I have been married for twenty-six years; in fact, we had just celebrated our anniversary on the day before I discovered the new lump in my breast. He had taken the day off from his job so we could have some fun together, with a nice lunch somewhere, and perhaps a bit of shopping. We ate at a fine French restaurant, but were disappointed because the food was not good and the service was poor. We had fun browsing the quaint shopping center, spending most of our time in a silversmith's shop where we bought a few tools and a sheet of silver for my own workbench. We enjoyed being together.

The day after our anniversary, we were invited to a small dinner party, in our honor, at our son and daughter-in-law's new home. It was to be after square dancing, because the entire family knows that we dance first on Friday nights, and other activities come second. Our son, Chip, works until nine o'clock in the evenings anyway, so we would gather for an elegant late supper about ten o'clock.

When we arrived, the house was beautifully candlelit, and Karen, our daughter-in-law, was busy in the kitchen, putting the final touches on the meal. Our daughter Laurie and her boyfriend, Mike, were already there, and there were kisses and anniversary greetings to us.

Food always tastes good to Tom and me after square dancing, but the food that evening was very special, warmed by the loving atmosphere we all felt.

"Karen, your potato soup is excellent," I said. "Is it from one of your gourmet cookbooks?"

"No, I just made it up," she replied, with pride.

I was especially proud of her because she had not been able to cook when she married Chip a year and a half earlier. They both beamed and accepted the compliments for the evening from each of us.

During the hour it took us to drive home, we spoke of our

three children and of the joy they have given us through the years. Ours had been an instant family, beginning with the birth of our first baby nine months and one day after our wedding, with the other two following within two years of each other. Our eldest, Priscilla, has been married for five years to Jack Rollins, a fine son to us and a real brother to Chip and Laurie. We always say that the nicest thing Pris ever did for Chip was to bring home a brother for him. He used to cry as a little boy and say to his daddy, "You and Mommie have each other, Pris and Laurie have each other, but I have nobody." Now he has somebody.

Pris and Jack are expecting our first grandchild in a few months, and, although they live the entire state of Texas from us, we are excited. Chip, our middle child, is the third generation of my family in the Oriental rug business, following in the footsteps of my father and brother. He looks handsome working among the beautiful rugs and seems to feel quite at home there. He and Karen look like brother and sister; both are blonde and blue-eyed and good looking in an unassuming way. We are glad that they are nearby, and we enjoy our visits with them whenever we are able to get together. Our youngest, Laurie, is a senior nursing major at Texas Women's, living at the dorm in the medical center here in Houston. The nursing program has been difficult for her, but she has persevered, and we have been her greatest fans. I know now from my own experience that she is a fine nurse, and I will never forget.

As we prepared ourselves for bed, I was amazed to see that it was two o'clock in the morning. I pulled my gown over my head and felt the lump on the side of my left breast with the inside of my upper arm.

"Tom, would you feel this lump?" I walked across the bedroom where he was sitting on the little needlepoint chair, which my mother had made and which I had enjoyed in the ten years she had been gone. "What do you think?"

"Oh, yes," he said. "That is different, isn't it?" He looked at me with concerned eyes as the room became very still.

We have been through much together, beginning with the very first months of our marriage. Because my first pregnancy resulted in toxemia and uremic poisoning, and the delivery was dangerous when Pris was born, we found ourselves separated for almost all of the first year of our marriage. It was a time of great testing for both of us, as I found myself being cared for in my mother's home while Tom continued his work in another town, joining me on weekends. It was painful for us because our time together is precious, and we still cannot tolerate separation well. From those early times of stress through all the years of raising our family, we had learned to depend very much on each other and, together, on the Lord. We had become extremely close. We knew instinctively that here was yet another time of testing for us. As always, however, we spoke to each other of our faith in the Lord, knowing that He would not give us more than He would expect us to handle.

I prayed that night for the courage to face the days ahead. I wanted to be able to place myself in the Lord's hands, so, even though I did pray for the best for myself, I knew that the Lord's will would be done. I remembered the words of the Apostle Paul who said that we are saved by our hope, and I was able to relax and sleep.

Even though I have had a history of fibrocystic lumps in the breast which have caused concern over the years and which have always before been unimportant, I knew immediately that this lump was different. My first action was early Monday morning, when I called for an appointment to see the surgeon. A time was decided upon for Wednesday afternoon.

After what seemed to me to be a brief and perfunctory examination, Dr. L. extended his hand to me and helped me to sit up, saying only, "This one is different, isn't it?" He left the examining room so I could dress. His nurse instructed me to join him in his office. I felt lightheaded.

He leaned back in his swivel chair and observed me over his glasses. "Now," he said slowly, "this lump needs to be removed right away. We need to see what it is. We'll do a biopsy while you are under anesthesia, and then we'll need to proceed according to what the lab report tells us." He explained quickly what different options were open to a surgeon, differences in types of mastectomies, and procedures that might be followed during surgery. He did not tell me anything that I had not heard before, or read in some of the women's magazines, but his words were blurred and jumbled in my ears; even so, I knew exactly what he was saying to me.

Then, suddenly, he leaned forward and looked straight into my eyes. "I wouldn't wait on this at all," he said earnestly. "If you were my wife, I would take that lump out right away. One or two weeks won't matter; however, I wouldn't wait a month or more." He sat back, waiting for my response. It made sense not to procrastinate, I agreed.

It is amazing how quickly these things can be arranged, over the phone, with even a few exchanged words of pleasantry. The surgery was scheduled for the following Monday, at one o'clock in the afternoon, and I would be expected to check into the hospital on Sunday afternoon between two and four o'clock, please. I would be given papers to sign stating my permission for the surgeon to operate as extensively as he found necessary; therefore, I should be considering, please, all the possibilities as he had explained them to me. He was patient and thorough, answering my few questions as they came to my mind, but he was also matter of fact and businesslike. I left his office dazed and just a bit sick to my stomach.

After shopping for a short time (looking for a robe for the hospital!), I picked Laurie up at the medical center as we had planned, and together we drove to meet Tom for dinner. We enjoy treating Laurie to a nourishing meal sometimes, because we know that nursing students are notorious for their poor eating habits! We enjoyed our meal together, talking of the next few days in which we would all be involved in the experience of my surgery. Laurie spoke reassuringly to me out of her concern as a daughter, with an added medical knowledge which gave me confidence. When we said good night to her at the dorm, I felt calmer.

Remembering with Paul that "the spirit helpeth our infirmities," and confident that "all things work together for good to them that love God," I prayed before bed that God would be by my side through this time as I had always known Him to be in every other experience of my life. And I thanked Him for that great blessing.

CHAPTER TWO

"BE CAREFUL FOR NOTHING; BUT IN EVERY THING BY PRAYER AND SUPPLICATION WITH THANKSGIVING LET YOUR REQUESTS BE MADE KNOWN UNTO GOD.

AND THE PEACE OF GOD, WHICH PASSETH ALL UNDERSTANDING, SHALL KEEP YOUR HEARTS AND MINDS THROUGH JESUS CHRIST."

Philippians 4:6, 7

We crossed the highly polished lobby of the hospital in the Medical Center; it shone in stark brightness. I followed the young woman who was my guide up the escalator to the second floor. She was black, and she was beautiful, with a smile and a cheery conversation that warmed my heart.

"That's your family with you?" she asked, with genuine interest.

"Yes, they came along to give me some support," I responded.

"That's real nice they could be with you." Smile.

She dropped me off at the blood lab on the second floor, wished me luck, and said she hoped that all would go well for me. I thought of what an asset she was to this hospital with that open spirit of concern.

Sitting down at the little table to give my arm to the lab technician, I was also able to look around me and take note of the other patients in the small lab. There was a large, older man who did not look too well, whose family had been allowed to accompany him up to the second floor. (My own family had been asked to wait for me in my room on the fourth floor.) His wife and another woman were sitting with him, along with a young boy about eight years old who was very curious about the pain of giving blood. He came over and stood right in front of me, questioning me over and over about my feelings as we both watched my blood fill the small vials.

For the first time, I noticed the petite blonde matron, obviously frightened and unhappy, who had become shrilly vocal concerning her feelings about herself and the hospital. She was beautifully groomed, and her clothes and coiffure were in the highest fashion, but her face and voice told the story of how she felt about this day. I was aware that I was staring.

She followed me into the spotless little bathroom where we were both to obtain a urine specimen.

"This place is filthy!" she called to me from her stall. "Look at all those paper towels out of place and fingerprints on the fixtures."

"Well, notice that the floor is really shiny bright," I offered in return from my stall. "The bathroom as a whole seems to be quite clean."

". . . and they give you this tiny bottle. . . . you're supposed to be able to collect a specimen. . . . going to report this to the hospital administration. . . ." she continued as I left to return my bottle to the waiting technician. I felt sorry for her, and, when I saw her again later, things had not improved.

After the electrocardiogram and chest X rays, I was guided to my room on the fourth floor for the first time. Tom was waiting for me, as well as Chip, Karen, and Laurie, all with lots of questions about the tests. The Medical Center was huge and impersonal, and I was happy to be with my family again. We had been together since early morning, attending church together and sharing our noon meal at the cafeteria, then driving to the hospital in one car. After a brief visit with one another, it was parting time, with Laurie walking back to her dorm, and Chip and Karen returning to their home. I had enjoyed the day with them, and I admit feeling a very real lag of spirit watching them go through the door. This was natural for me, because, although I am not a "smother" type, I do like and enjoy my children; they are my closest friends.

I looked around the room for the first time. It was a bright and cheery room, but strange in shape and design.

"Queer room!" I said to Tom, who was already reading the Sunday paper. "It's chopped up and 'cater-cornered,' and that means all the furniture is oddly placed." I thought that this was certainly going to be offensive to my artist's eye. Tom was unimpressed.

"Put your gown on and get ready for bed," he suggested, still reading.

"But it's only five o'clock!" I protested. "I'm not sick."

"Well, you'll feel more comfortable if you get out of your clothes, and you will need the rest." Now he was looking up at me, and I did as he suggested. That's the way it is with us!

We each had a chair and were enjoying the newspaper when our pastor, John Craig, knocked and pushed open the door. Looking up through the blur of my reading glasses, he could have been my father coming through the door; the coloring was the same, the receding hairline, and even the expression and demeanor were similar. Only I perceived this, and the little flicker of remembrance was gone in a moment. The three of us sat in a tight cluster near Tom's chair, because the room offered few choices. I sat on the edge of the bed, and we spoke of my surgery the next day.

"Well, it's to be a biopsy, and, while I'm under the anesthesia, the lump will be sent to the lab for identification. Depending on what they find, Dr. L. will continue the surgery," I explained as it had been explained to me.

As we talked, a young nurse known as "Kelly" came in with the very papers that I was to read and sign concerning my surgery. I needed to understand all the aspects of breast surgery, as well as the different types of mastectomies, and then sign the papers giving permission to the surgeon to perform the surgery indicated by the lab report. I had no desire to return for a second round of surgery, so, after a few questions to Kelly and some thought, I signed the papers.

We visited a bit after Kelly left us, with Tom and John enjoying some conversation about square dancing, which they both love, teasing each other about whose left foot is the more contrary! Then the three of us stood in a small circle, holding hands, and John offered a prayer for me and for Dr. L., asking God for strength for the patient and skill for the surgeon. "In every thing by prayer and supplication with thanksgiving, let your requests be made known unto God . . . and the peace of God, which passeth all understanding, shall keep your hearts and minds. . . ." His prayer brought the presence of the Lord into the room, and my spirit was calm. I was grateful.

Shortly after the minister left, Tom had to leave as well; the evening chores awaited him, and he would be alone to take care of them. Moreover, there were the animals at home, Maggie, the dog, and Cre-Cre, the cat, who would be hungry and eager to be fed for the day. We don't tolerate separations well, and this night was no exception. Each of us made the classic effort to uphold the other as we held hands and said good night. He kissed me and turned away from the bed, walking quickly out of the room. Watching him go through a few tears, I knew, above all, that he would be praying for me, too.

Again I turned my attention to the room. I couldn't believe that the color was predominantly orange! I thought of what an awful color orange was for me, wishing for my favorite blues and greens, which are so much more becoming to me. Even the bed-spread was a terrible orange! Well, I was certain that some women just love orange and would be delighted with this room. To the right of the bed was the large orange leather chair that could open into a bed, where Tom would sleep the night of my surgery. The air conditioner was just above and the full length of that chair, so whoever sat or slept there would be terribly cold. The window was right above the air conditioner and rose the entire height of the wall, with nondescript draperies of orange and brown that hung open limply. I had a view of the building tops in the Medical Center, drab in the evening haze. There were several combinations of lights, and I tried them all until I was satisfied with the brightness of the room.

When Kelly came in to say good night to me, I felt another wrench, because she had already become a friend. She was very young, cute, and blonde, and obviously loved being a nurse.

"I'll be back tomorrow, darlin'," she called over her shoulder as she turned toward the door. "Good luck tomorrow in surgery."

The night nurse was a large black woman, Jefferson, who had the prettiest face I think I'd ever seen—lots of compassion there. She did her job efficiently, taking my vital signs, bringing extra blankets, and getting the room ready for the night. She told me to call her on the intercom if I needed anything during the night. I liked her at once.

I didn't need anything during the night, but Jefferson came into my room several times just to check on me. I refused the sleeping pill that was offered to me, saying that I would have no trouble sleeping unless I took the pill, in which case I would walk the floors all night long. That wasn't going to happen to me tonight. Several times during the night, however, Jefferson opened the door and called to me, "Mrs. Munroe, Mrs. Munroe. . . ."

Sleepily, I turned my head toward the door. "Yes?"

She called back, "Are you cold, Mrs. Munroe?"

"No, I'm fine, thank you, Jefferson."

"Well, if you need anything, just call me. Have pleasant dreams now." I loved that. She always ended her nighttime rounds with me by telling me to have pleasant dreams. I did sleep well, awakened by the early morning nursing shift.

My surgery was scheduled for one o'clock in the afternoon, and I really dreaded the wait of the entire morning. When I had told Dr. L. that I was sure to go into surgery with a headache without my coffee, he had given permission for me to have one cup of coffee. About midnight, as she rustled about the room, Jefferson mentioned that I was not to have anything by mouth from then on. I was wide awake in a flash!

"Oh, no, dear, I'm having coffee in the morning, and Dr. L. has given his permission." I would have fought for that.

"Well, if the doctor said it's okay."

The morning nurse, Joyce, who was a woman about my own age, was friendly, capable, and helpful. She had heard of the coffee, and brought me a cup, looking very much like the cat that had the canary. Joyce mentioned that cup of coffee several times afterward, and I knew she realized how much it meant to me.

During the long morning hours, my sister-in-law, Maryann, came to be with me; she is a registered nurse who ministers at the bedside of any in the family who needs her. She is a mighty nurse, as I knew from previous experience. She settled all her bags and bundles in the proper places, and then she pulled out the white doctor's coat that gave her the final touch of authority. She then settled herself in for whatever the siege might be for me, and I felt better just seeing her there. Laurie, too, came to take her place beside the patient, who also happened to be her mother.

Moments before I was to receive my preoperative shot, Charles Miller, our associate pastor, came briefly to say that the prayer chain at our church was in progress for me. Then he read from a small card a prayer of healing for me: "The Lord is my healer, I shall not fear. . . . Yea, though I pass through sickness and suffering, I will fear no evil. . . . Surely healing and mercy shall follow me all the days of my life. . . . I will abide in the love of the Lord. . . ." I was comforted by the promise there.

Tom arrived about the same time as Joyce, bearing the preoperative shot, and she ordered everyone out of the room. Dutifully, Tom and Charles turned to leave, followed by Maryann and Laurie, looking over their shoulders at me with questioning eyes. They were not happy at being asked to leave.

"Joyce, those last two are nurses, too, you know," I said quickly.

"Oh, I didn't know," she replied. "Come on back in."

It wasn't long before my mouth began to go dry, and reality started to slip away, but I remained conscious until I was taken into the operating room. Tom was holding my hand, and Laurie and Maryann were assuring me over and over that they would be praying for me. How I felt the strength of those assurances.

"Thou preparest a table before me in the presence of my troubles; Thou annointest my body with healing power; my cup of joy overflows."

CHAPTER THREE

"THE LORD BLESS THEE, AND KEEP THEE;
THE LORD MAKE HIS FACE TO SHINE UPON THEE, AND BE GRACIOUS UNTO THEE;
THE LORD LIFT UP HIS COUNTENANCE UPON THEE AND GIVE THEE PEACE."

Numbers 6:24–26

The young man who came in to transport me to surgery was gentle and kind. He lifted me ever so easily from the bed onto the rolling cart, with a soft, calming conversation directed just to me as we struck out into the wide halls. I was fully aware of where we were going: first onto the elevator, then through great double doors into the window-lined halls of the operating rooms. The young man continued his soft chatter the entire trip, telling me about leaving Florida and coming to Houston, and now trying to adjust to life in the large city. Asking questions, I was making a feeble attempt at concerned conversation as well as offering encouragement to him. He pulled my cart over against the wall and said good-bye, adding that he hoped that I would do well in surgery. I appreciated his genuine concern.

I lay there, my heart racing, waiting for whatever would happen next. A nurse in green scrubs walked briskly over to me and, taking my chart from under my pillow, she asked if I were Mrs. Munroe.

In my condition, she's asking if I'm Mrs. Munroe, I thought weakly. *Shouldn't she know that I'm Mrs. Munroe?*

I told her that I was Mrs. Munroe, and she asked again, just to be sure, I suppose, that I really was Mrs. Munroe. I assured her again that I was.

"Your heart is racing," she said, checking my pulse. "Are you frightened?"

"Yes, of course I'm frightened!" I responded, feebly. Foolish question.

About that time I was wheeled into the large white operating room, into position under a giant honeycomb of lights above me. A group of nurses, masks in place over their faces, were coming and going, each busily doing her job. Often one came over to where I lay motionless to check the patient, and, with only their eyes showing above the masks, I remember thinking that they all had beautiful eyes. I suppose that if one spends the better part of her working day behind a mask with only her eyes showing, she makes the most of her eyes! It wasn't only well groomed, artfully made-up eyes that I was noticing. There was interest, concern, and intelligence.

A very young anesthetist had gotten hold of my arm and was trying to get it into position for the injection into my hand. He had a narrow kind of shelf that pulled out from the table that could be maneuvered into different angles, and he struggled with that shelf and my arm until he finally found the proper combination. When he pulled my arm too high, the bursitis in that shoulder began to cause me pain.

"Am I hurting you?" he asked, anxiously.

"Yes," I answered, "that's my bursitis shoulder." I was amazed that he would care. *The Lord is my shepherd; I shall not want. . . .*

Then he began the painful process of trying to locate the vein into which the anesthetic I.V. would be inserted. He tried several times, each time more painful than the last, before he was able to begin the injection. He murmured over and over that he was so sorry to cause me this pain, and I could only moan my response.

My final memory of the operating room is the intense burst of light from the honeycomb above me, and Dr. L. standing nearby, hands upheld in the traditional pose of surgeons, scrubbed and ready for surgery. He was looking up and seemed aloof from the hurried activity of the others near me. I prayed one last silent prayer, asking the Lord's blessing on me.

Only later did I learn of the different dramas that took place while I was in surgery, and I was interested to hear them all. After I had been wheeled out of the room, Maryann asked Tom to offer a prayer for my well-being and, holding hands, the three of them prayed quietly for me. Then Tom bolted from the room and made his way down to the chapel. He was desperate to make connection with the Lord, but, as he told me later, he was in such a frantic state that he couldn't calm down enough for the Spirit to enter his heart. Picking up the Gideon Bible that lay before him, he searched the pages and began to read. From Philippians, the fourth chapter, he found the peace he needed in the passage that encourages us to take every worry to the Lord in prayer and supplication.

As he continued to read, he was further comforted by these verses from the book of Paul's letter to the Romans:

"Likewise the Spirit also helpeth our infirmities: for we know not for what we should pray; but the Spirit itself maketh intercession for us with groanings which cannot be uttered . . . and we know that all things work together for good to them that love God. . . ."

This was precisely the message he so urgently sought, because, although he wanted to pray, he had not been able to let go of his fears and allow God's peace to enter instead. He continued reading from that eighth chapter, began to feel the calming of God's love, and found his fears subsiding.

". . . If God be for us, who can be against us? . . . who shall separate us from the love of Christ? . . . nay, we are more than conquerors through Him that love us. For I am persuaded that neither death, nor life, nor angels, nor principalities, nor powers, nor things present, nor things to come, nor height, nor depth, nor any other creature, shall be able to separate us from the love of God. . . ."

What a promise! Believing that promise, Tom relinquished his fear and put his hand in the hand of the Lord. He was anxious to relate all this to me as soon as I could understand.

My dear friend Pat Thompson found Tom in the chapel, studying the portrait of a donor that hangs there. She had heard at her circle meeting that morning of my impending surgery and was very upset by the news.

"Why wasn't I told?" she asked with some agitation. Pat does have a tendency toward agitation. I love her.

"There wasn't time, Pat," Tom explained.

"Well, I heard about the surgery this morning at circle meeting," she replied, "and there was such a lot of misinformation about it. I was so worried about Liz!"

Tom told her what he knew would be involved in the surgery, and, after a brief visit, he walked outside with her to her car. He promised to call her as soon as there was anything to report.

I had my own circle meeting at my house during the few days between my visit to the doctor and going to the hospital. Our circles are small groups of Christian women, perhaps twelve or fourteen, who meet on a weekday morning to study the

Bible, pray together, and enjoy one another's fellowship. On the Thursday before I entered the hospital, I carried out the plan for my circle to meet in my home, and I told these dear ladies about my surgery. Here were some of my best friends, and I felt great relief in sharing this burden with them. Each one assured me of her prayers; in fact, we all prayed for my well-being right there within the circle in my living room. ". . . where two or three are gathered together in my name. . . ." His promise was to be there in our midst. I believe that.

Of course, I had called to tell Pris and Jack about the impending surgery, and also my brother, Richard, and his wife, Vickie, in San Antonio. I wrote to my maiden aunt in New York to say that I was going for a biopsy on the lump in my breast, really to alert her to the fact of my problem. Aunty Dickie is a retired schoolteacher, my mother's only sister, and very close to our family. She is a dreadful worrier, and I knew she would take the news of my surgery hard. I was right; she did. To the two or three friends I spoke to the few days before surgery, I mentioned that I was going into the hospital, and I told John and Naomi Craig at square dancing, because their prayers would be important to me.

In the two or three days remaining before I entered the hospital, I had been busy getting my house in order, preparing some simple foods for the freezer, and doing some hurried Christmas shopping. I talked with the children several times, and they impressed me with their staunch, supportive attitudes. Pris wondered if she should make the trip from Lubbock, but, since she was almost seven months pregnant, I did not want her involved in this stressful situation. She assured me that she and Jack would be in constant prayer for me, and I was convinced that they would be. She told me later how difficult a time it had been for her, hundreds of miles away from her mother in surgery and wishing to be at her bedside. I truly missed her, too.

Some time after I had been taken into surgery, Dr. L. came into the room where Laurie and Maryann were waiting. He told them that the lump he had removed from my breast had been analyzed in the lab and been found to be malignant. He would need to do a modified radical mastectomy.

"Oh, can't you just remove the lump?" Laurie asked, hopefully.

"Now, that wouldn't be a cure, would it?" he answered patiently. "Your mother has already signed the permission papers, but I wanted to let you know what we are doing. Find your dad and give him the information, please."

Both Maryann and Laurie knew that Tom had gone down to the chapel, and each hoped the other would see him first to break the news that Dr. L. had just released. Neither one knew that Tom had found peace during his time in the chapel and now would be the strength of their little group. Laurie went down to the chapel and, missing her dad, assumed that he had gone to the room, where Maryann would relay the doctor's message. Instead, she met him in the hall as she emerged from the elevator and tearfully told the news of my mastectomy. When she broke down into tears, her father reassured her.

It was after six o'clock in the evening before I was wheeled back into my room, although I was unaware of time at that point. My first memory after surgery was the same as all my first memories post-surgery . . . vomiting! I always came from the still, dark world of anesthesia back to the real world vomiting, and this time was no different. I remember that Maryann and Laurie took turns holding the pan and wiping my mouth as I strained my head to the side and retched. Kelly came in several times with the bedpan saying, "Can't you tinkle, darlin'?" Then she took her turn at holding the vomiting pan, murmuring over and over, "Poor little darlin', poor little darlin'. . . ." I marveled at her compassion. She had just put me on the bedpan for the third or fourth try when our pastor, John Craig, came into the room. I was in that early post-anesthesia consciousness in which I was slowly becoming aware, could hear and feel, but was unable to open my eyes or speak. I felt his hand on my forehead and heard him speak the familiar blessing from the Old Testament:

"The Lord bless thee, and keep thee; the Lord make His face to shine upon thee, and be gracious unto thee; the Lord lift up His countenance upon thee and give thee peace." He patted my head and left the room. I felt an instant uplifting from this ancient blessing, and I nodded my recognition of it. I also felt my mortification at my position on the bedpan, but I felt sure that ministers saw that all the time, and were not easily rattled by what they encountered in hospital rooms!

Outside the door, Laurie was talking to Naomi Craig and was able to reassure her that I would be all right.

"Mother has a great faith, Mrs. Craig. She'll be fine," she

said. They hugged and comforted each other. When Laurie related this episode to me later, I could only think: "See how these Christians love one another. . . ." The longer I live, the more truth I perceive in that.

Chip and Karen had come to my bedside, and, although I did not see them, I heard Chip say over and over, "We're praying for you, Mom; we're praying for you." I nodded my understanding and my thanks. Tom had taken his position for the night on the awful orange chair, now changed into the awful orange bed. He said later that each time Jefferson had come into the room, he had had to jump out of bed and fold the lower part out of her way, finding on remaking the bed that the foot had sunk lower and lower to the floor. He never made the offer to sleep there again.

Jefferson came into the room every hour during the night, taking vital signs, helping me to the bathroom, and taking her shift at the vomiting pan. In the middle of the night, I spoke my first words since surgery to her: "You have the prettiest face I've ever seen," I said, in all sincerity. She thanked me and went about her business with a big smile. Every lady likes to hear that she is pretty.

An offensive sound was becoming intrusive, and, opening my eyes for the first time, I was stunned to see that Tom was watching a football game! The sound was quite low, but, in that strange room, the TV was directly over my head, and the very idea of football was causing some weak response in my nonfootball heart. Our children had always been involved in band, high school and college, and being the participating parents we were, we went to many, many football games. The more I saw, the more I disliked. Now as I became more aware, I thought to myself, *Oh, is there nowhere on earth that I can be free of this game?* I turned my head slowly on the pillow, closed my eyes, and drifted off again. At least it was good for Tom to have this diversion . . . maybe it even helped to make the orange bed more acceptable.

CHAPTER FOUR

"FOR WE KNOW THAT, IF OUR EARTHLY HOUSE OF THIS TABERNACLE WERE DISSOLVED, WE HAVE A BUILDING OF GOD, A HOUSE NOT MADE WITH HANDS, ETERNAL IN THE HEAVENS. . . . FOR WE THAT ARE IN THIS TABERNACLE DO GROAN, BEING BURDENED:

THEREFORE IF ANY MAN BE IN CHRIST, HE IS A NEW CREATURE: OLD THINGS ARE PASSED AWAY; BEHOLD, ALL THINGS ARE BECOME NEW."

II Corinthians 5:I, 4a, I7

In the unreal world of post-anesthesia darkness, I was filled with a sense of real peace, even though I knew by the feel of tight bandages on my chest and my arm that the mastectomy had been accomplished. No one had to tell me that. What I did not know, however, was that my chest muscles had not been removed; I had undergone a modified radical mastectomy in which only my breast and the chain of nearby lymph nodes had been removed. Tom explained this to me later when I was better able to understand, and I was uplifted by a profound sense of relief. The Lord does truly work in mysterious ways; I am more than ever convinced of that wonder.

Two thoughts persisted in floating in my mind, quite subconsciously, I am sure, because they presented themselves at almost the same moment when I became aware that the mastectomy had been accomplished. My senses had not yet fully recovered, I was not speaking or opening my eyes, but I was thinking and feeling. I was curious about the meaning of the word "MASTECTOMY," knowing what it meant now for me, of course, but anxious to understand the derivation of the word. Why was this surgery not called a "mammectomy," I wondered, since other terms relating to the breast use the root "mammo," terms such as "mammogram." At home later, Laurie and I looked up the word in her medical dictionary and found that the derivation was from the Greek word *"mastos,"* which means breast. That was resolved.

The other idea that floated about in my darkened mind was not so easily resolved. Through no conscious thought of my own, with sudden clarity, the idea presented itself that I should write about this experience from which I had not yet even fully awakened! Here would be a way that I might be able to witness to the fact that in every experience of life, no matter how devastating, God is present and working in the lives of those who trust in Him. I already knew from first-hand, personal experience that God reveals Himself to us in every crisis of life, as well as in our moments of highest joy. There is a peace and calm in life's shattering times that can come only from the love of God, whose promise has been to be with us to the ends of the earth.

When my mother died, only six weeks after my father's death ten years earlier, I was in greater shock and grief than I had ever known before. We had been to her home late at night and, providentially, found her lying on the floor of the den in a deep coma, from which she never awakened. I prayed for strength and courage, asking the Lord to be with me in some very real sense, because I had never had a greater need. I found comfort walking in the little rose garden in the backyard of my parents' home; the roses that Mother had tended so lovingly bloomed profusely the seven days she lay unconscious in the hospital, and each day we were able to cut and arrange beautiful bouquets for her room. As I walked in the garden on the day of her death, I was stunned to see that every bush was drooping, every bloom was dead . . . except for one mighty bloom! The one remaining blossom was the most perfect specimen, the largest rose I had ever seen; it was glorious shades of pinks and reds, growing Heavenward on the tallest, thickest stem in the garden. Thanking the Lord for such a loving reminder of His constant presence in my life, I had to stand on a stool to reach for that magnificent rose, which I cut for all to enjoy.

Throughout my life, there have been many experiences when I have felt in a very real and positive sense the hand of the Lord extended to me, and reaching myself in faith and gratitude, I have known the peace that does indeed pass our understanding. And so, as I came back into reality after this surgery, once again I felt that that same calm peace was mine; however, this time was different. Now I was feeling a very positive nudge toward expressing what I know from my own experience of God's love, His caring for each of His children, and how accepting that love on faith enables us to recover from life's most devastating experiences. I was compelled to tell what I knew, and from there I could trust in the Lord to do as He would with it.

Often as I wrote these words, I became discouraged and, putting my head down on the typewriter, I told the Lord that I didn't think I could do this! Although I was a creative person and I sketched and painted, writing a book had never been even a remote area of interest to me, but I was committed and I would persevere.

The outflowing of love and concern for me following my surgery and all the prayers in my behalf were heartwarming and uplifting. I was feeling the immediate strength that came from the prayers of my family and friends, and I thanked God for each one. Flowers and plants were crowding into the tiny room, and cards were brought to me every day. Laurie's boyfriend, Mike, came in with the first arrangement of flowers, and after that it was a real challenge to find a place for anything else. Friends and family came and went, and it seemed that I was never alone.

Cyndi Tifft came early in the morning of my first post-operative day, and, leaning over the bed, she whispered her greeting to me.

"Why are you whispering, Cyndi?" I asked in a little whisper.

"Well, because you are whispering," she replied. We both laughed.

I had asked the young resident that morning why I had no voice, and he told me that my vocal chords had been affected by the tubes inserted into my throat, and it would be some time before they returned to normal. The same young resident was curious as to why I was still vomiting twenty-four hours after surgery, and when I told him that I was sensitive to pain-killing drugs taken by mouth, that they always caused nausea and vomiting, he ordered that the injections for pain be stopped. For twenty-four hours I had been receiving injections for pain, coupled with injections for the vomiting, and now, late in the afternoon of that first post-operative day, the vomiting stopped, and I was able to tolerate small sips of liquid. Did apple juice ever taste better?

Dr. L. checked on me several times a day, always examining the position of the hemo-vac, and tugging at my arm to see how the muscles were coming along. His instructions to the nurses about the hemo-vac were very precise, I suppose, because he had been instrumental in introducing this method of drainage into this hospital. Too, he was more concerned about the exercise of my arm than he was about the pain I was suffering in that arm. I described the pain in my arm by likening it to an imaginary medieval torture device of heavy cast iron, lined with millions of tiny sharp needles; once clapped onto my arm very tightly, the screws were then tightened more and more. When I mentioned this horror story to the young resident, he responded by telling me that there had been dissection in that arm and so, of course, there would be pain. . . . "Dissection?" That was sobering!

I was going to the bathroom on my own steam, but the nurses were still measuring my output there, as well as the drainage, which was collected each day in the hemo-vac. I was sitting up a bit by the evening of that first post-operative day, and I began to make noises about having breakfast the following morning. The rainbow of gelatins that had been offered tasted like cotton in my mouth, and the broths had made me ill, so small sips of juice had been my only nourishment since I had last eaten on Sunday. Early Wednesday morning found me sitting up in the orange chair, eagerly awaiting breakfast. My heart sank when the aide delivered her tray with the usual juice, jello, and broth, and I became a trifle hysterical, ringing for June, and yammering in a childish way: ". . . I'm dying of starvation . . . the doctor said that I could have something to eat. . . . I need food . . . the doctor said. . . ." I could have cried.

"What would you like to eat, honey?" June asked, sympathetically.

"I don't care what I eat," I ranted, "just something solid. FOOD!"

After the longest fifteen minutes of my life, the young aide returned, this time bearing a tray of glorious scrambled eggs, bacon, toast, and coffee. I began to eat with gusto, but after two or three bites, I found myself full; however, I determined not to waste this precious food. Cyndi came to sit with me for a few moments and, slowly, as we chatted, I was able to eat all the food on my tray. "Waste not" was my motto that day. Richard, my brother in San Antonio, called, too, during my milestone breakfast, and this was our first chat since my surgery. He was very concerned, and Tom had kept him informed. He and Vickie called often, and I was always cheered by our conversations.

Maryann came to sit with me each day, and when Tom and my brother-in-law, Alec, arrived after work, the three of them could have supper together. Laurie, too, came every day, sometimes leaving for a class, then returning to visit awhile longer. She was like a real breath of fresh air. Pat Thompson came to see me every day for a short visit, and I was always refreshed by her presence. My friend, Barbara Carmichael, brought me an enormous coloring book from Caryn, her four-year-old, who was one of my Sunday School pupils. It would make a fine project for my class of four-year-olds, providing I could refrain from coloring the huge mural scenes before I returned to my class!

Some of Laurie's nursing friends were stopping by to visit me for a few moments, instructing the nurses to be very kind to me, because I was their friend's mom. Our pastors came often, reading a brief passage from the Bible and always leaving me with prayer, the pause that lifted and refreshed. The love and concern of Christian friends, as well as the loving support of my family, were some of God's blessings to me in the hospital.

Through all this, I noticed that Tom was trying very hard to be the genial host to one and all in the hospital, and I was disturbed by the effort he was making to be his usual, strong, effervescent self. He is by nature a witty and outgoing person who enjoys people and loves to create fun and laughter, but knowing that he was suffering with me, I wanted him to know that he need not continue this pretense because of me. One evening, when we were alone, I asked him to sit by my bed so we could talk; he took my hand through the bars, and we enjoyed a few quiet moments. I spoke to him of what was in my heart and mind, trying to convince him that he was not expected to behave as though nothing had changed in his life. He was allowed to feel the same emotional stress we were all experiencing, and he could lower his defenses a bit to show his own feelings. He relaxed visibly and began to speak what was truly in his own heart.

"Well, I've been thinking of the important things in our life together," he began, "and I realize that nothing has changed because of your surgery. The most wonderful part of all this is that we still have each other! I didn't marry you for your body; I married you for who you are. I still have you, and all the things that we've enjoyed together, we can continue to enjoy. Our life together has always been first with us, and that hasn't changed. We can continue to enjoy our children, and our grandchildren; we can travel and camp together, and we can still have fun with our friends and family, as we have always done. Life will not be changed that much for us. I love you, and I thank God that I still have you with me."

I was moved and warmed by his declaration, and have felt throughout my convalescence that same spirit of loving support; he could not have been a more loving or supportive husband. If

I became discouraged or despondent during the weeks following my surgery, Tom would have none of it.

"You're doing fine, Charlie," he'd insist. "No time to be downhearted—you're doing too well now!" A loving mate has to be one of God's richest blessings, I do believe.

Thanksgiving was my third post-operative day, and on my breakfast tray that morning I noticed not only an especially nice meal, but also a lovely greeting from the hospital administrator. He wished all the patients a happy Thanksgiving, saying that, although this was not the ideal place to spend the holiday, if each patient thought hard enough, there would surely be cause for thanksgiving. I was touched and impressed by his message, and I recalled and appreciated it all day long. It had already occurred to me as I began my slow walks around the nurses' station and could see patients so much worse off than I, that I had much for which to be grateful. I had lost a breast; I could see a patient who had lost both legs. I thought of her this day and prayed for her and for myself, that I should not forget the proper thanksgiving for all the blessings that were mine.

Laurie and Tom brought turkey and dressing from our favorite cafeteria, and we three feasted together. Laurie complained that, of course, it was not like Mother made, but it was shared, and that made it delicious. Chip and Karen had gone to a family reunion and came in later to regale us with tales of kith and kin in east Texas. Pris and Jack called to wish us a happy day and to say they missed us. The feeling was quite mutual. More family came for a short visit, including Alec, who had drawn a Thanksgiving cartoon for my door. It was a picture of a huge Thanksgiving bird, roasted and waiting to be carved by a surgeon with knife and fork held high, with the nurse standing by holding a bowl of cranberry sauce. It was fun and imaginative, causing much comment in the hall, and we all enjoyed it.

Sleeping at night in the hospital had become impossible, but not for the obvious reasons. True, the nurses were in and out all night, and my bed was a real disaster; the mattress seemed to be constructed of layers of old newspapers, bundled and tied into neat packages, covered with a matted pad, and topped with a slickly starched sheet. My arm was arranged on several thicknesses of stiff hospital blankets, and my head was about the only movable part of my body. What was really disturbing my sleep, however, was a strange tickle in my throat that awakened me every time I began to doze off and that was accompanied by a brief, violent nightmare. Jefferson brought me juice to soothe my throat, but the cough persisted. Often in the middle of the night I gave up the notion of sleep and read from several books I had with me. One was a beautiful book of photographs from nature, which looked like impressionistic paintings; each one was illuminated with passages from Thoreau. I studied the photographs and read the text, savoring the book as I had never been able to do before; I had never been able to give it an entire night's attention before.

Then, as I often do, I opened my Bible, too, letting it fall open at random, trusting the Lord to find there some message for myself. Several times, in those long nights on that tough hospital bed, the book fell open to the fifth chapter of II Corinthians. Here the Apostle Paul speaks of our bodies as earthly tabernacles in which, while we are at home here on earth, we are absent from the Lord. He speaks of the burdens we will bear in our earthly bodies, and of the new bodies that will be ours when we are at home with the Lord. My body had just borne a heavy burden, and I was eager to read further:

> "For we know that when this tent we live in is taken down . . . when we die and leave these bodies . . . we will have wonderful new bodies in heaven, homes that will be ours for evermore, made for us by God himself . . . these bodies make us groan and sigh, but we wouldn't like to think of dying and having no bodies at all . . . our aim is to please him always in everything we do, whether we are here in this body, or away from this body and with him in heaven."

It seemed right to me that I should read what Paul said of our earthly bodies. I relaxed and slept awhile.

CHAPTER FIVE

"CONSIDER THE LILIES OF THE FIELD, HOW THEY GROW; THEY TOIL NOT, NEITHER DO THEY SPIN: AND YET I SAY UNTO YOU, THAT EVEN SOLOMON IN ALL HIS GLORY WAS NOT ARRAYED LIKE ONE OF THESE. WHEREFORE, IF GOD SO CLOTHE THE GRASS OF THE FIELD, WHICH TODAY IS, AND TOMORROW IS CAST INTO THE OVEN, SHALL HE NOT MUCH MORE CLOTHE YOU, O YE OF LITTLE FAITH?"

Matthew 6:28–30

Some good can come from every experience in life. ". . . and we know that all things work together for good to them that love God. . . ." I had lots of thinking time during the five days that I lay in the hospital bed, contending with emotional recovery as well as physical. I felt strongly that the Lord had a message for me in this shattering interruption of my life. It was as if I had been stopped in my tracks, thrown flat on my back, and now, with my very existence at intermission, I was able to quietly ponder some of life's deepest verities. I felt the need to take advantage of that time.

I had a great husband and, with our family raised and gone from home, we still *liked* and enjoyed each other. We had loved and respected our parents as long as they lived, and our memories of family were good ones; we had all enjoyed marvelous family gatherings, fun with aunts, uncles, and cousins, times which we were able to recall with happiness and laughter. We had been children involved with our parents and participating parents with our children. Looking back brings no regrets, no bitterness or recriminations. We have a circle of good friends, some of long standing, and have still been able to enjoy new friends as our life together progressed. Although we had shared some devastating tragedies in our twenty-six years as a family, we had always been upheld and sustained by the love of God. We had each learned to trust in Him, and we had that hope of which Paul speaks in Romans. Our Christian conviction has always been strong, and faith has been the driving force in our lives. Tom and I had both grown up in the faith, and we had decided before our first child was born that we wanted our children to share that faith. We decided that ours would be a Christian family, and we trusted that the Lord would give the direction for that purpose.

Now, as I lay on my back in the hospital, I knew that more was to be required of me. Primarily, I felt that some changes were to be made in my spirit of giving, of being more understanding, kinder, and more loving to others. When I mentioned these thoughts to my family, Chip quickly said, "Gee, Mom, you're already the sweetest one I know . . . except for myself, of course!" I laughed, and Chip, ever the clown, was pleased. Seriously, I know that real giving never ends. One must never rest in extending herself to others; the old feeling of "I've already done my share" just is not valid. Now, in fact, I was thinking that my share had not been enough, that no one was ever able to give enough.

The dilemma was to discover the means whereby I might be empowered to become a more loving and giving person. I knew already, of course, that such power can come only through the strength of God through Jesus Christ, and I resolved right there in the hospital that I would "pray without ceasing" for that strength. My prayer life should become much more intense, my study of the scriptures should increase, as I know that to be the greatest source of strength, and my own Christian witness should become more dynamic. None of these ideas was new to me; however, now I had a fresh attitude toward them. Perhaps the writing of this book was an example of new force in my life, another way to extend myself. Maybe it would only serve to reinforce and revitalize the new attitudes that had been such a vital portion of my thinking in the hospital. I never wanted it to slip away from me.

Second, the decision to take better care of myself, to stop pushing myself to exhaustion, and to slow the pace of my life was an attractive resolution that I was able to make in the hospital. Being a hard worker is an inherent trait in my Armenian blood; I come from hard-working stock! My parents were both immigrants from Turkey to this country, making me first generation born in America, and they had dreamed of opportunities awaiting them here. They were not only willing; they were eager to work and struggle to provide all those opportunities for their family, and no honest labor had been beneath them. My father had been a college graduate who spoke five languages, but his first job in this country was picking grapes in the California vineyards. My mother was so anxious for the education denied her that, when her children had left home, she had herself tutored in math in order to get her high school diploma, and then went on to college. What a history to live with! With this background, my brothers and I never balked at hard work; we didn't dare.

I had always admired the prudent woman in the book of Proverbs, who rose while it was still night, who spun and weaved, and who toiled willingly for her family. She was of such value to her husband that he had no other needs in life:

> "Strength and honor are her clothing; and she shall rejoice in time to come. She openeth her mouth with wisdom; and in her tongue is the law of kindness. She looketh well to the ways of her household, and eateth not the bread of idleness. Her children arise up and call her blessed; her husband also, and he praiseth her."
>
> Proverbs 31:25–28

Can anything in life be of more value to a woman than a husband who praises her and children who call her blessed? Greater than rubies, indeed. I realize that I worked too hard at the menial chores that all women know well, but I had never resented even the unpleasant tasks, because home and family had been too important to me; even with a master's degree, I always felt that my place was in the home, and that my education served me well right there. I had no problem with liberation because I had never been enslaved! Now I was able to see that my health might be affected by the relentless pursuit of the clean house, the sparkling glassware, and the crisp linens, topped off with being the fresh, scintillating wife and mother. I knew what was important to me, and my new resolve was to pursue only the truly valuable concerns as they existed for me. I was going to take better care of myself.

The other idea that became a resolve in the hospital is humorous in a way, but fraught with serious meaning to me. I am a chocolaholic, and I might have broken the chains that bound me to my addiction! I had been addicted since early childhood, and there were many funny anecdotes in the family, relating to my affair with chocolate. Tom brought several boxes of chocolate to the hospital, ostensibly for the nurses, each one larger and more tempting than the last. One by one, the boxes were opened, sampled, and savored by everyone except me. I was not tempted. Food was just beginning to taste good to me, and the sight of all that chocolate almost made me ill. Therefore, on Thanksgiving evening, as Tom (the ringleader!) with Laurie, Chip, and Karen joining in the fun, sat by my bed, right under my nose, and gorged on chocolate candy, I saw too clearly what a gluttonous group giving vent to their appetites looked like. At least two boxes were open, one on Laurie's lap and one on Chip's, so the four of them were in a tight cluster, the better to reach and grab the candies.

"Have you tried this one?" someone would ask.

"Take a bite of this one," another added. "It's marvelous!"

Each one had candy in both hands, another piece in the mouth, with all eyes glued to the remaining pieces in the boxes. Their mouths were so full that their speech was slurred, but the orgy continued. I turned my head away to avoid the entire scene and told myself that if this is what I had become (and I knew I had), then I would have to change that habit. I did not renounce chocolate entirely; however, I wanted to be able to eat just one piece of candy at a time, no more. When I told Pris of my resolution, she said, in all earnestness, "Gosh, Mom, you were our teacher. It won't be as much fun without you." I felt worse than ever.

The Lord was speaking to me in many ways in the hospital, and I was paying attention. Above all was the distinct feeling of peace and well-being that came of the knowledge of God's presence with me, his love and concern for me, and the calm spirit that was mine, right there in the hospital. I knew that friends and family were praying faithfully for me, and those prayers were sustaining me throughout this ordeal. I told Pat that I was amazed at how calmly I was accepting my situation, and I was certain that the prayers in my behalf were responsible. Tom had said that he had tried many times to send his prayers on their way, but the Lord had had to put him on "hold," because there were already so many prayers in my behalf!

"I certainly hope the prayers don't stop now, because if they do I will really come down with an enormous thump," I told Pat during one visit with me. This peace and joy that comes with believing in the love and mercy of our heavenly Father does indeed pass understanding.

Cards and letters were arriving each day from friends and family, every one an inspiration and delight to me; some were from friends around the country, writing to sympathize because they had undergone mastectomies years ago and were just fine now. That was marvelous to hear. Friends whom I loved and admired, many from my church fellowship, wrote their encouragement, telling me that I was much in their thoughts and prayers. Over and over, the words were: ". . . We're praying for you. . . . We're praying for you. . . . ." I knew that was true, because I felt the effect of those prayers, and I was very grateful.

Of all the cards I received, the most touching came from Pris's dearest friend, Melody. The card contained a passage from the book of Matthew, which is full of meaning to me, the heart-warming words from the Sermon on the Mount:

> "Consider the lilies of the field, how they grow; they toil not, neither do they spin: and yet I say unto you, that even Solomon in all his glory was not arrayed like one of these. Wherefore, if God so clothe the grass of the field, which today is, and tomorrow is cast into the oven, shall He not much more clothe you, O ye of little faith?"

Added to the quotation from Matthew already printed on the card, written in Melody's distinctive handwriting were the words from the last verse of that sixth chapter:

> "Take therefore no thought for the morrow: for the morrow shall take thought for the things of itself. Sufficient unto the day is the evil thereof."

Then, in her sweet way, she wrote of her prayers for my recovery, for strength for Tom, and of her love for our family. Tears filled my eyes.

Dr. L. came in to see me at least twice a day, normally sitting a few moments to answer questions or even just to chat. Always, he pulled at my affected arm to note improvement in muscle ability, causing me pain, but he did impress upon me the importance of the exercises he had shown me to regain the use of my arm. I understood him, and I was following his instructions. On the day before Thanksgiving, he came into my room with a large grin on his face, more pleased than I had ever seen him before. He said that he had been breathing down the necks of the lab people to get a speedy report on the eighteen lymph nodes that had been removed from under my arm during surgery. Obviously pleased, he said that, of the eighteen nodes, only one had been found to be involved (cancerous), and the prognosis was most favorable if three or fewer nodes were involved.

My spirits were already good, but this news was a real boost. I asked when I might go home, and he seemed relieved to tell me that I could go whenever I wanted to! Together, we decided on Friday morning; I could hardly wait to go home.

My body was very sore, and not in the area of surgery alone. Every muscle had been affected by the retching I had done, and then further aggravated by my efforts to spare the more painful ones, as I struggled to get in and out of bed. I told Tom that I felt as if a truck had run over me! Although I was moving about more easily and was growing stronger each day, every movement caused pain. My arm, which was tightly wrapped with elastic bandage from wrist to shoulder, caused the greatest pain, but I exerted the effort to continue the exercises. My chest was heavily bandaged from the middle of the chest, under the arm to the back area, with the heaviest concentration of bandages over the drainage tubes, which still hung from my ribcage. The hemo-vac swung from my body like a small purse, tied around my waist with package string; it was a nuisance, but Dr. L. would not remove it for another week.

The tissue in every part of my body surrounding the bandages was black and blue, which I knew meant hemorrhage under the skin. This I could understand, and Dr. L. assured me, too, that it was quite normal. Altogether, it was not a pretty sight. I tolerated the physical appearance of my body, devastated as it was, because, I was certain, I had the strength promised me to meet every circumstance of my life. Too, I remembered the lilies of the field, and I was calm.

CHAPTER SIX

"UNTO THEE WILL I CRY, O LORD, MY ROCK; BE NOT SILENT TO ME, I BECOME LIKE THEM THAT GO DOWN TO THE PIT.

HEAR THE VOICE OF MY SUPPLICATIONS, WHEN I CRY UNTO THEE, WHEN I LIFT UP MY HANDS TOWARD THY HOLY ORACLE.

THE LORD IS MY STRENGTH AND MY SHIELD; MY HEART TRUSTED IN HIM, AND I AM HELPED: THEREFORE MY HEART GREATLY REJOICETH; AND WITH MY SONG WILL I PRAISE HIM."

From Psalm 28

Friday morning was interminable; I wondered if Tom and Laurie would ever come to take me home. My mistake had been to leave my bed at about six o'clock in the morning, before the sun had even risen over the tops of the buildings. I stood at the sink to take a mini-bath as I had done for a couple of days, brushed my hair, and attempted to apply a bit of makeup. I tucked a yellow daisy into my hair, and, feeling rather stunning, I sat in the orange chair to await the arrival of my breakfast tray. I was engulfed by pillows and several layers of folded blankets, my bandaged arm resting on one mound, my sore back supported by another. The young girl with the breakfast tray finally bustled into the room, took one look at me, left the tray, and hastily made her retreat. She remembered my hysterics of that first morning when I needed something to eat! I ate the meal slowly because of the butterflies in my stomach. I was going home.

The nurses who had been my friends were all off for the weekend holiday, and the new shift knew that I was going home. No one was even interested in my vital signs, certainly not in my comfort or emotional state. The family and friends who had been faithful visitors would see me at home, so, for the first time in the hospital, I felt all alone.

My plan had been for Laurie to pack my personal things and for Tom to gather together the books and plants, but now I decided to do my own packing. The real challenge was to consolidate into the small bag I had brought all the extra items that had accumulated during my hospital stay, working at a slow pace, and with a wounded wing at that! On the walls Laurie had tacked up colorful Thanksgiving decorations and fall leaves to brighten my room, and I stretched mightily to recover each one; they had been purchased at some sacrifice for her, I knew, and I wanted her to have them for her own home. After the flowers and plants had been gathered into one area of the room, I was exhausted. I should have gotten back into the bed. Instead I sat back in my nest of linens and began to read my Bible.

A very young girl came into my room and asked perfunctorily, "Are you going home today?" After I told her that I was surely going home today, but before I had a chance to say anything more, she quickly turned on the television and began to strip the bed of the sheets. She looked to be about sixteen and several months pregnant, and she was immediately engrossed in the soap opera she was watching over her head as she worked. Knowing that she wasn't interested in conversation, I tolerated the sound from the television, and went back to my reading. She worked so slowly that, after about fifteen minutes, she gathered up all the sheets and towels and left for the room next door, and the next installment of her program. By now I was longing to return to my bed, but she had left it with only a rubber sheet on top of the mattress. (I should have known that a rubber sheet was hiding under the lumpy pad, over the stacks of newspapers!) Happily, I was able to get comfortable with all the bedding I had propped up around myself, because it was afternoon before Tom and Laurie finally came for me.

"Where have you two been?" I fairly yelled, as they came in . . . smiling. "I was so worried about you and I'm cold . . . no sheets on the bed . . . and I WANT TO GO HOME!!!" I was sounding like a brat again. They both stared at me, waited until I had finished my tirade, then explained that they had enjoyed a leisurely breakfast together and had simply lost track of time. When they told me that they had also cleaned the house for my homecoming, I pulled myself together and forgave them. After all, how many did I know who were willing to clean my house?

A cute young nurse, Gwen, helped Tom load the cart, and then pushed me in the wheelchair out to the waiting car. Her eyes were wide and brown, and they filled with tears as she told us that her mother was coming into the hospital next week to have a mastectomy; I assured her that she would be the same comfort to her mother that Laurie had been to me. We told her to be sure to pray for her mother as well as nurse her, and we promised that we would be in prayer for her, too.

The world was strangely bright and busy, and I was fearful and insecure in the noise and frenzy of the freeway traffic. Coming into the quiet serenity of our home was a blessed relief, and I felt real life and spirit returning to my heart as well as my body. I lay on the sofa in the den, watching as Tom unloaded the bags and plants, and Laurie prepared our lunch. My cup was overflowing.

Chip and Karen joined us that first night at home, bearing a smoked turkey from Karen's family as well as other goodies for our dinner. With some instruction from the bedside, Laurie planned a wonderful meal, especially delicious to one who had been on hospital fare for several days! She brought a tray to my bed, where I was content to eat and listen to the conversation from the breakfast room. Although my appetite was not good yet, the remembrance of those first bites of lovingly home-cooked food is still marvelous. Having been unable to sleep my last several nights in the hospital, I was exhausted and utterly drained. I was anxious to turn out the lights for the night, confident that, now that I was home in my own bed, sleep would quickly come. By the time Tom came to bed, I had dozed off many times, only to be awakened by the same irritating tickle in my throat, accompanied, as in the hospital, by the brief nightmare. I ached to turn from my back, but even the slightest movement to either side was painful, so I remained on my back, struggling with discomfort and fatigue. As the night wore on, I became more exhausted and discouraged, until, finally, awakened by one last terrible nightmare, I left the bed to go into the bathroom.

Tom raised his head as I made my way across the room.

"Are you all right?" he asked.

"I'm okay," I answered. My voice trembled and tears stung my eyes. He was right behind me in a moment, turning on the light and holding out his arms to me. I collapsed against his chest and cried.

"What's wrong, dear?" he asked gently. "Are you in pain?"

"Yes, I am in pain, and I'm so tired but I can't sleep again. That same tickle in my throat keeps wakening me, and I'm having those nightmares. I'm just worn out," I cried.

He held me until I was quiet and then led me back to the bed. Maybe the cough syrup he offered soothed my throat, or the tears had eased my tension, or perhaps it was just the tender, loving care; I am not sure. I did sleep.

For about a month following surgery, I was uncomfortable during the night, and sleep was difficult. I went to bed in a real cocoon of blankets and pillows, fluctuating between too hot and too cold. The pain in my arm was constant, the medieval torture device still at work! Now I was beginning to suffer hard pain in the incision area, and, because I don't tolerate the pain medication well, an occasional aspirin was all I used for my pain. The drainage tubes had begun to pull at my flesh under the heavy bandages, and any movement became excruciating, twisting that sword in my side. At times, I felt pain in the missing breast, understanding for the first time that this is what amputees must feel in a missing limb. I guessed that severed nerves were going wild trying to adjust to the trauma of surgery.

Even the bandages encompassing my body caused distress. Dr. L. had warned me that the bandages would become blood-stained as the drainage tubes pulled away the flesh, and they would begin to have an odor. They did just that, and I was repelled by the odor. We didn't dare to change the doctor's dressing, so Tom simply inserted more clean squares of gauze under the soiled bandages to catch the drainage overflow. I began to feel as though I had grown another appendage under my night-gown. Looking back on those first weeks post-surgery, I do not wonder that I was unable to sleep.

My solace in the night when I was unable to sleep was to slip into the kitchen where my Bible lay on the breakfast table, fix myself a cup of tea, and lose myself in stories from the Old Testament. More than any other food, I was enjoying the *katah,* which Pris had made and sent to us. Katah is an Armenian bread, very rich and buttery, difficult and time-consuming to make, which Pris makes better than her mother, or even her grand-mother, who was our teacher. When nothing else tasted very good to me, this *katah* was delicious. Reading, my heart was inevitably lifted by my excursions into the ancient past of my own faith, and, after an hour or two, I returned to bed to sleep a bit.

Laurie was providing the greatest of nursing care, more nurse than daughter when the occasion demanded, and always with that loving concern that was her natural attribute. It occurred to me that her four days at home during the Thanksgiving break were just another of God's blessings at this time in my life. She was cheerful and gracious in all the chores she assumed; in addition to taking care of me, she was cooking for the family, washing and cleaning, and performing all the tasks that were normally mine. My bed was changed each day while I took my mini-bath and changed my gown, and there were always fresh surprises to cheer me and brighten my room. With all this, she was even trying to study! I was amazed at her energy and stamina. We laughed at her remark about all the work involved in keeping a home; then she said, "I'm not sure that I want to get married . . . too much work!" Going back to school would be a rest for her.

Before she left for school on Monday evening, Laurie emptied my hemo-vac as she had done every night we had been home.

"Mother, I'm concerned that the drainage output is so many more c.c.s than it has been since you came home from the hospital," she said, tying the cord in place around my waist. "Be sure to tell the doctor when you go tomorrow to have the tubes removed."

Her eyes were all concern as she led me back to my bed. I thought of all the many nights that I had tucked her into bed and heard her evening prayers, and, now, here she was, tucking me into bed. I hated to see her go, and I felt the tears welling again. Mike had come for supper and was going to drive her back to the Medical Center. Tom walked them to the car, and, when he came back to the bedroom, I was in tears. We wept together.

My disappointment was terrible when Dr. L. said on Tuesday that he felt he could not remove the tubes because of the heavy drainage of the night before. The trip into town had been an exhausting one, so my energy was at a low ebb. Just the effort of getting this bandaged body in clothing, something big and baggy, soft and warm, had been overwhelming. I carried a small pillow from home, fearful of my bad arm and painful chest, and I was afraid that Dr. L. would not approve of my protecting my arm this way. He understood. He told me to come back on Thursday, and he would remove the tubes at that time. I agonized at the thought of this exhausting trip into town, all for naught today, to be repeated day after tomorrow.

Friends and neighbors, as well as faithful Maryann, were coming and going each day; it seemed as though a conspiracy were afoot that I should not be left alone. All sorts of good food was brought in, and Tom especially relished all the goodies. Wonderful as I know him to be, he cannot cook at all; I often accuse him of not even being able to butter his own bread! Any "cooking" he was doing at this time was done under my supervision; I would sit in the kitchen as he followed my instructions. It wore both of us out, but we were good-natured about it. He liked to say that he married me because he admired the fact that the old-country men in the family appeared to be "head of the house," with the women apparently serving in happy submission. Of course, it was not that simple, but I knew that the reason Tom couldn't butter his own bread is that I had always done it for him!

The daylight hours were easier for me because my friends were in and out, gifts and flowers were delivered, and my phone rang constantly. Tom made a spot for the phone on the bed within easy reach of my good arm, so, when my friends called, I was always able to chat. The sun shone through the double windows of my bedroom each afternoon for several hours, casting its healing warmth over my body, and I relaxed comfortably in its rays. It sent golden light radiating through the stained glass hanging at the window; the panel was my own design, a large descending dove worked in yellow and pale greens, and the brilliance of the sun filtering through the colors never failed to cheer me. I often fell asleep for short naps, watching the play of shadows on the dove, feeling warm and at peace with the sunlight spreading over me. I used these times for short prayers, thanking the Lord for increasing strength and asking Him for endurance to tolerate the pain, which was such a difficult part of the day.

The time of the most excruciating pain came on the second Thursday after my surgery, eleven days after, to be precise. Tom and I returned to Dr. L.'s office for the removal of the drainage tubes. The trauma in the tissues of the area had caused me to run a high fever, and I was weak and weepy, in no condition for the drive into town and unprepared for the pain to come. The removal of the bandages caused me to flinch; then, when Dr. L. leaned over me and in one swift effort released the tubes from my flesh, I simply was not able to restrain my cries of agony.

"Well," he said, quickly depositing the odious culprit in the wastebasket, "the good book says to do what you have to do quickly!"

He offered his hand to help me sit up, and, through my tears, I said, reproachfully, "That's not biblical." He looked at me in surprise and reminded me of Jesus' command to Judas when He was betrayed. He was right, of course, but the correlation eluded me here. A doctor friend, Elizabeth Senekjian, explained to me later that the drainage tubes were anchored into

the body by sewing them through tiny holes in the tubes directly into the flesh to be drained. Small wonder that I howled!

For two days I remained in pitiful condition. When Richard and Vickie called from San Antonio, I was unable to hold the phone, and Tom had to prop it up on my pillow; however, the effort to speak was too great, and I stopped trying after that conversation. I thought I had reached my lowest ebb . . . but more was yet to come.

Just as I had begun to recover from the feverish debilitation of the last three or four days, I began that most dreaded of maladies, a migraine headache. Tom and I had wondered that I had not been afflicted in the two weeks since my surgery, but now here it was. It started early in the evening, quickly developing into the intense, mind-numbing pain that never relents. It was accompanied, as always, by the violent vomiting that continues for hours until all the stomach fluids have been extracted. No treatment had ever relieved either or both of these symptoms for me, and even injections given in the doctor's office had failed to bring relief. I was unable to cope with this further agony, and I sat on the edge of the bed, moaning softly and holding my head in my hands. No longer able to sit still, I wandered aimlessly about the house, followed by a frantic Tom, desperate to know how to help me. Dr. L. suggested a suppository medication, knowing that I could not tolerate anything by mouth, but that intense vomiting reflex did not allow sleep. I continued throughout the night in my agony.

I thought of the Psalmist who, overwhelmed by his affliction, cried out for the Lord to hear his prayer:

> "Hide not thy face from me in the day when I am in trouble; incline thine ear unto me . . . my heart is smitten, and withereth like grass. . . . my days are like a shadow that declineth . . . but thou, O Lord, shall endure for ever. . . ."

My days of anguish had come and I wondered if I could have tolerated my physical and emotional distress without the certain knowledge that my prayers were heard, that God was with me, and I would endure.

As I began to recuperate, I was disturbed by the fact of my cancer, a sure condition verified by the lab report at the hospital. Dread thoughts came and went, and I decided, rather than assume a cloak of bravery, to give vent and conversation to my fears. I read articles and pamphlets on cancer, especially breast cancer, hoping to educate myself; I spoke to my cousin, Schuyler Aijian, a pathologist in California, about my prognosis and further therapy. and he was an immense help to me; I spoke to friends, some of whom had had mastectomies like me, some who had suffered other cancers, and we compared treatments and conditions. Conversation was real therapy. One precious friend, Alma Stoltje, who had come through her own bout with cancer five years earlier, came to me bearing a warm, fresh apple cake and these very wise words: "Elizabeth, you just go on; you just go on. God will take care of you, so you just go on!" That had to be the best advice I could have heard, and knowing that Alma had done just that, I felt I would be able to, also.

Sue Newman called early one morning, asking if it was too early to call to say simply that she loved me.

"Sue," I responded, "it's never too early to say 'I love you!' "

"Well, I want you to remember that your surgeon saved your life," she told me emphatically, "and you must be grateful for that—don't forget." She spoke of her surgery several years ago, and I especially appreciated her positive attitude. It was contagious.

My neighbors were thoughtful and concerned, calling often with offers to run errands or go to the grocery store, and coming in with surprises or food for our next meal. When Emily Michaud and her darling little girls came bearing our entire meal, salad through dessert, I was truly touched, knowing in my heart that their kindness would never be forgotten. Throughout these first few weeks at home after my surgery, I was aware that the love and prayers of so many faithful friends and family were still sustaining and upholding me, and I thanked God for them all. Although I am still keenly aware of my condition, my fear has subsided and I have simply decided to "just go on." God is my enabler.

CHAPTER SEVEN

"FOR OUR LIGHT AFFLICTION, WHICH IS BUT FOR A MOMENT, WORKETH FOR US A FAR MORE EXCEEDING AND ETERNAL WEIGHT OF GLORY;

WHILE WE LOOK NOT AT THE THINGS WHICH ARE SEEN, BUT AT THE THINGS WHICH ARE NOT SEEN: FOR THE THINGS WHICH ARE SEEN ARE TEMPORAL; BUT THE THINGS WHICH ARE NOT SEEN ARE ETERNAL."

II Corinthians 4:17–18

There was one important bridge yet to be crossed before the climb to recovery could begin . . . the patient needed to face herself in the mirror, stripped of masking bandages, and accept the image she found there. Using every possible excuse, this patient procrastinated for over a week. When Dr. L. had removed the stitches two weeks after surgery, he had lightly taped a thin gauze bandage over the incision area, padding the drainage openings with heavier protection because the wounds were still draining. I used those bandages as my security blanket, not yet ready to see what the surgeon's skill had wrought to my body. I longed for a real bath, to feel the hot water wash over my sore body, just to enjoy a clean, fresh scent about myself. Since I was unable to bathe with the bandages still in place, I continued the mini-baths at the bathroom sink, meticulously avoiding the bandaged areas.

When the soiled gauzes needed changing, Tom led me to the bed, where he changed the bandages for me. I was simply not ready to face myself. I shall never forget, however, that he was able to care for me so gently, and that he was willing to face my disfigurement before I was able to accept it myself, all the while encouraging and boosting me! That is the kind of love of which the Apostle Paul speaks in his letter to the Ephesians, exhorting a man to love his wife as he loves his own body, loving her as he loves himself; and that is the kind of husband a wife can revere and to whom she can submit in love. I shall not forget.

Dr. L. had given permission for me to shower just three days after he had removed the stitches, and Tom suggested several times that probably the light bandage over the incision was no longer necessary.

"It looks real good, Charlie," he said often. "The incision is healing, the holes from the stitches are closed, and the bruises are fading. Do you want to skip the light bandage?"

"Oh, well, I feel more secure with my chest covered," I replied, rationalizing to myself as well as to Tom. He understood and joined me in this little charade as long as it was necessary.

I was not troubled with depression or self-pity during the weeks following my surgery; perhaps I thought often of my fellow-patient in the hospital who had lost both legs. I was not at all sure that a breast was important enough to grieve its loss. There were too many blessings to be counted, too many friends and loved ones pulling for me, too much to anticipate now to allow myself to become bogged down in despondency. That kind of energy could be better used in the positive thinking that would enhance my recovery.

I remembered, too, that Paul, in all the dire circumstances of his life, through the kinds of travail that most of us will never experience, said: ". . . for I have learned, in whatsoever state I am, therewith to be content. . . . I can do all things through Christ which strengtheneth me." I am able to identify with such an attitude because the Armenian people have a history of persecution and affliction; however, their strength in the Lord has been their strength to endure. From my father, who had known such affliction, I had learned to persevere, and now this time of pain and debility I found could be endured. Still, the bandages remained.

The elastic wrapping around my arm was a real source of discomfort. Dr. L. had shown Tom how to unwind it to clean my arm, give it a light massage, then rewrap the arm from shoulder to wrist. We did this several times a week, and I found some relief from the constant pressure I felt under the wrapping. We were stunned that the arm was so thin and shriveled, and the skin so flaky. Although my upper arm was quite numb, the pain there was persistent, and that seemed a contrary combination. After six weeks, when the wrapping was removed, we began a measuring ritual, which I understood would be important for the remainder of my life. I have suffered only minimal swelling in my affected arm, but I am aware that I must be cautious about trauma or infection to hand or arm, because lymph-node-fighting capability is absent there.

One bright morning, I decided to remove the bandage from my chest as I was taking my daily mini-bath, standing at the bathroom sink before the room-sized mirror there. The adhesive tape gave easily under my gentle tug, first the two strips extending across to the opposite breast, the two reaching under my arm around to my back. As the bandage fell away slowly from my body, I eased timidly into the sight facing me in the mirror. The image there was very unattractive, but, blessedly, I felt neither shock nor revulsion. I happen to have a real collection of scars from my head to my toes, so the sight of another wound to my flesh was not the devastating surprise it might have been. This scar was an angry red, and it stretched in one horizontal line across my left chest, ending well to the back of under my arm. I had heard several tales of two scars, or of scars that extended from neck to waist, so I was unprepared for a scar that I knew wouldn't show under my clothes. There was still swelling, and the line was most irregular with dips and curves; there was discoloration with puckerings and depressions. No clean line here! As a seamstress, I think I had expected a neater look. I looked only briefly this first time, knowing that time would improve the image and my acceptance of it; this was a real milestone, however, and I was profoundly relieved that I had passed it.

When my dear friend Dr. Elizabeth came to visit on my second weekend at home, we talked about the surgery and the resulting disfiguration; she helped me in many ways, putting to rest some of my doubts and fears as only a knowledgeable friend can do. Besides that, she cleaned my house and ironed Tom's shirts, and that is a true-blue friend! Later, at another time, we made Armenian food together, wherein four hands were better than two, and that is a true Armenian friend. Sitting and visiting, sharing coffee and goodies together, and feeling the loving concern of such dear friends had to be a very important phase of my recovery.

Jeanne Wilson, a special friend who came to spend the day with me, had always been an inspiration because of her Christian dedication and strength of character. As we visited, she spoke of her young son, lost many years ago in an accident, and of her daughter, totally handicapped, who had died only recently. I have marveled at the love and devotion of all the years that she and Marion had faithfully expressed to their child, and their greatness of spirit was an example to me. Once again, as we enjoyed the day together, I drew strength from her. When her car did not want to start at suppertime, Tom and I were delighted that she could share our meal. Her witness was beautiful to behold, and we were refreshed.

"Watch, thou in all things, endure afflictions, do the work of an evangelist, make full proof of thy ministry."
II Timothy 4:5

That is Jeanne.

When Naomie Craig came for the day, she came bearing great sacks of food, but she also brought what she called "spiritual food" for the nourishment of our hearts. These were several tapes of Bible studies, led by a dynamic young preacher, which she knew would strengthen and sustain me. I was missing my usual church experiences, and, since it would be two months before I could participate in the Sunday morning services, I did indeed appreciate the spiritual refreshment I received from those tapes. Naomie and I talked of our families, our mutual delights and concerns, the fun and excitement of anticipating our first grandchildren, and always at the core of life, the blessings that were ours in our faith. Before she left Naomie tucked me in for my afternoon nap, and, sitting on the little loveseat by the bed, she read to me from the book of Isaiah until I was relaxed and ready to sleep. Her gentle spirit brought comfort and solace to me.

"Never flag in zeal, be aglow with the Spirit, serve the Lord."
Romans 12:11

That is Naomie.

Because my exercises were going slowly, and my arm just didn't want to stretch much above my waist, Laurie became anxious that I have the overdue call from a volunteer in the "Reach to Recovery" program, which is sponsored by the American Cancer Society. In this remarkable program, the volunteers are women who, having recovered themselves from mastectomies, call on women who have just undergone the surgery, and from their own experiences are able to encourage and assist the new mastectome in various ways. Within a few days of Laurie's call, a lovely lady came to visit me; bringing with her a most helpful book written by the woman responsible for starting the Reach to Recovery program after her own mastectomy. She also brought a little bag of exercise aids, which she demonstrated, one by one. She was such an attractive lady, fresh and vital, with obvious zeal in the enjoyment of life, that I was heartened by her visit.

I hope to be one of the volunteers in the program when my time arrives.

She had also brought a very soft stretch bra and some dacron fluff to fabricate a lightweight prosthesis, which might suffice until I would be able to tolerate a heavier, genuine prosthesis. For three weeks after surgery, I had been unable to wear any type of bra, preferring to dress in loose gowns and robes, mainly because nothing would fit over the bandages without causing pain. I wore a 34D bra, so the things I chose to wear were full and gathered over the bosom to conceal the disparity that was apparent there even with the bandages; after the bandages were removed, the difference was greater.

My cousin Joyce, who called from Pennsylvania often, told me of her mother-in-law's great attitude following her mastectomy.

"Gosh, Liz," she said in all earnestness, "Mother just tucks a couple of tissues into her bra, and that's all she's ever done." I chuckled at the sight of me, 34D on one side and a couple of tissues on the other!

"Well, Joyce," I laughed, "perhaps a pair of Tom's gym socks, but tissues? No, dear."

The soft, stretch bra with the dacron fluff was funny, too. The shaped form looked like a football and, combined with the other breast, which was pretty well flattened by the stretch of the bra, the difference suggested that the mastectomy had been performed on the opposite breast. Instead, I created something for myself which was exactly what I needed until my chest had healed enough to tolerate a prosthesis. I chose an old bra, all stretched out of shaped, but big and soft, and pinned into the cup a form made from a white hankie folded over a likely amount of the fluff. I thought my creation was just fine, and I enjoyed wearing it long after I brought home other kinds of prosthesis.

I was in no hurry to leave the security of my home or to struggle to get myself dressed and leave the comforts that were mine; first, I was still in pain and happier to stay close to the bed, and, too, I was weak because strength seemed slow about returning. I was content to be able to get through the day with its small activities. I was beginning to assume the responsibilities that Tom had been performing for me, especially the cooking, which delighted him. I could handle the washing and drying of our clothes, folding and putting things away, and I was beginning a little cleaning and dusting. I needed to use my arm, and I was glad to be feeling more useful every day.

I was also excited about this book, and each day gave creative time and thought to this project. My family was supportive here, too, encouraging me and cheering me on by reading the pages as I completed them, even helping by offering their ideas and suggestions. Pat, who is a former English teacher, and whose use of the language is excellent, was kind enough to promise that she would read the first rough draft and use her red pencil to correct it as she would with one of her students. After reading the first four chapters of my book, Pat called to say that she liked what she had read.

"If your purpose in writing this book has been to tell how God has been your strength, together with loving support from your family, through this experience in your life," she said sincerely, "then I think you have succeeded." I was delighted to hear her say as much, and I told her that was exactly what my purpose had been, thank you!

There is a passage of scripture that is full of meaning to me, which has been in my heart for many long years; at a time in my very young life when I had reached a heartbreaking turn in the road, I prayed earnestly for direction, waiting for the Lord to guide my way. When my thoughts and feelings were most confused and unhappy, I pulled from a small box of Bible verses, right from the middle of the full box, this verse from Paul's letter to the Corinthians:

> "For our light affliction, which is but for a moment, worketh for us a far more exceeding and eternal weight of glory; while we look not at the things which are seen, but at the things which are not seen: for the things which are seen are temporal; but the things which are not seen are eternal."

My heart was touched by this message to me, which seemed to come from the Lord just for me, and I was enormously strengthened at that time in my life when my need was great, and those verses remain ones that still enable and empower me all these many years later. I prayed, and the Lord heard. His goodness and mercy have continued through the days of my life, and my most recent crisis has only confirmed and reinforced my belief.

CHAPTER EIGHT

"HAST THOU NOT KNOWN? HAST THOU NOT HEARD THAT THE EVERLASTING GOD, THE LORD, THE CREATOR OF THE ENDS OF THE EARTH, FAINTETH NOT, NEITHER IS WEARY? HE GIVETH POWER TO THE FAINT; AND TO THEM THAT HAVE NO MIGHT HE INCREASETH STRENGTH.

. . . THEY THAT WAIT UPON THE LORD SHALL RENEW THEIR STRENGTH; THEY SHALL MOUNT UP WITH WINGS AS EAGLES; THEY SHALL RUN, AND NOT BE WEARY; AND THEY SHALL WALK, AND NOT FAINT."

Isaiah 40:28–31

Christmas was coming, and with it the anticipation of family gathering with all the tradition that is ours as a family. I wanted desperately to keep our time together as normal as possible, with the same fun and fellowship we had always enjoyed; however, with a mother who was having difficulty just shuffling from the bedroom to the kitchen, it was going to be hard to share a normal family get-together. I was determined to try!

First, I was going to have to get my body going, no small task. Every muscle was sluggish and troubled, bones aching and stiff, and I wondered how even to begin an exercise plan. Amazingly, my back, for the first time, didn't cause much trouble, and Tom and I were both surprised that it remained strong and able. There was, however, one very unwilling left arm, as well as two stiff, sore legs and hips, and I found it almost impossible to move into my old routine of morning exercise. I was determined enough to continue and, noticing that each day brought some improvement, I was encouraged to persevere. My rewards came when I was able to extend both arms out to my sides and twist my body very carefully, and when I could bend from the waist and reach gingerly for my toes.

The next step was to stretch out on the floor to do the lying-down exercises. I struggled to ease myself down, but found that the effort to get down (and hopefully back up?) was already exertion enough, and it was days before I was able merely to lie down on the floor. The day did come, finally, when I could lie face down on the cushion of the bedroom rug and hesitantly raise arms and legs simultaneously. I shouted, "HALLELUJAH!" right out loud, praising the Lord and giving thanks for physical capacity returning.

> ". . . They that wait upon the Lord shall renew their strength; they shall mount up with wings as eagles; they shall run, and not be weary; and they shall walk, and not faint."

What an amazing promise that is!

Excited about my returning strength, I began to plot my schedule for the two weeks left before Christmas. Although I had put away a few gifts before I went into the hospital, there was still much to be done. I had fabric that had been waiting for my traditional Christmas sewing, and I hadn't known, of course, that I would be disabled just when I should be sewing. Now I wondered if I dared begin. I reasoned with myself, and I won. This kind of creative outlet would be good for me, therapy for my arm, and the gifts were needed under the tree for all three of the girls. So it was that, two weeks home from the hospital, I began to cut and sew again. It was too soon.

I had chosen teal blue corduroy for a matching skirt and vest for Karen, and it went together well. The pattern was a simple one, although actually I felt, after making and lining both pieces, that I had sewn three garments. I tried the skirt on for length and, satisfied, I pressed them and folded the suit into a gift box. I should have stopped then, but I continued.

The heavy corduroy I had chosen for Pris didn't seem right, somehow, and I was already tired of sewing on corduroy and couldn't face all the lint that it created. I was really tired of sewing but unwilling to admit that.

"Tom, how do you feel about running me down to the fabric shop?" I asked one evening after supper. He looked at me as though I were not quite bright; I was in my robe, only dressing to go to the doctor's office, and had turned down any suggestion to go for a ride or out to eat.

"Are you up to going shopping?" he asked. He didn't think that I should even sew at all. I had three days remaining in my sewing week, and he knew I was pushing myself, even if I did not.

As I browsed through the fabrics, I chastised myself and thought that I needed to have my head examined for this stupid venture. My head was swimming, and I felt weak and ill, thinking that I was going to pass out right there in the store! I chose my materials quickly, calling for help when I was unable to lift the bolt of fabric. I was determined to complete this project, and, now that the materials were at hand, I would begin tomorrow.

My evening jaunt had tired me, so the next morning was not very productive. Although the heavy blue cotton moved effortlessly under the sharp scissors, the effort of the cutting alone exhausted me. Still, I pushed. The sewing machine took on the appearance of an ogre, and I longed to put it all away, never to sew again, but I continued. When the garment was almost complete, I sat on the little loveseat in the bedroom to put the finishing handwork on hem and sleeves. I was cautious about pricking my fingers with the needle, as I had been warned in my Reach to Recovery booklet, but, because I was tired, of course, I did stick the needle into my finger . . . several times.

"Okay, Liz," I told myself, "time to quit. You can push yourself again in the morning." I scolded myself for beginning to show signs already of the old me, so soon after my resolution to be more calm and take life more slowly. I soaked my wounded thumb in hot water, then rubbed antiseptic cream into the reddened spot to discourage infection. It worried me.

I was elated the next morning to be finishing the job and so excited by my very last stitch, that I gave the same thumb a wicked jab in the sore and reddened spot. I was stunned to think that I had so injured myself on that final stitch, and, fatigue and fear combining, I began to sob, tears flowing freely. I stood at the bathroom sink, sobbing loudly and soaking my thumb in hot water. I could see infection already starting, and I was afraid.

"Oh, where is Tom when I need him?" I cried. "I'll just have to call him and tell him what a terrible experience I've had. . . . No, that's childish . . . but I need him. . . ." As I reasoned with myself and the tears calmed me a bit, the phone rang. Amazingly, it was Tom!

"What's the matter, dear?" he asked, sensing in the way a husband of many years can, that there was trouble. What a torrent I unleashed over the phone.

"Well," I sobbed, "I just stuck my thumb in the same place, right under the cuticle as I did yesterday, and it's bleeding. . . . I was finishing . . . my very last stitch. . . . I hate to sew; I'll never sew again . . . sick of the sewing machine . . . poor thumb. . . . I'm scared. . . ." All this jumble of words was further garbled by my wailing and crying. He listened sympathetically.

I was so relieved by this call when I needed him that he was able to talk to me and help me to a calmer state of mind. How did it happen that he reached out to me when my need for him was the greatest? Haven't we been told that God does good things for us, that he knows our every need, that even the hairs of our heads are numbered? From the book of Matthew, we read:

> ". . . For your heavenly Father knoweth that ye have need of all these things. But seek ye first the kingdom of God, and his righteousness; and all these things shall be added unto you."

If I had not believed before that this was true, now I would be convinced.

This outburst was the last overwhelming emotional release of my recovery period and the one that most relaxed my physical tension, as well as fear of wounds to my affected hand. I will not forget that my hand is vulnerable, and I will protect it as far as possible, but I have accepted the fact that hands will be hurt, all caution notwithstanding. Surely, a leather glove would be useful in my silversmithing. I remembered cuts, bruises, and burns sustained for my craft! I couldn't stop creating, I decided. For now, however, I was simply delighted to have completed two unique Christmas gifts within the allotted time, and pride in this accomplishment was an important step in the road to recovery. Creating anything is marvelous therapy.

There were to be two more shopping excursions before our Christmas gathering. One was to a nearby store for Laurie's gift; the other, one week later, was to the grocery store. One cold Saturday morning, three weeks home from my surgery, still in bandages and no bra, found me bundled into a bulky sweater and baggy slacks on the busy road to the stores. Tacky!! Tom had driven me, taken me by the arm, and holding me up literally, supported me about the store. He was no better looking than I, with his old leather fisherman's cap and his shabby Saturday work clothes, so we found that we were pretty well ignored by the salesgirls. Strength did not allow for any browsing at all, so the first garment I touched was what we chose, and we were on our way back home in just minutes. Certainly not what one could consider an exciting shopping spree! Now I was relaxed, at least, to have the proper collection of gifts under the Christmas tree.

Our next venture, to the grocery store, just one week before Christmas, was on Saturday morning again. The stores would be jammed with shoppers, and I vacillated between sending Tom with a mammoth list and going myself to shop with his support. The memory of the brief jaunt through the fabrics was too fresh, and I grew weak remembering.

"I don't think I can make it," I told Tom as we were leaving.

"Well, just give me the list, and I'll go to the grocery store," he said. "I can get all the things you'll need for your Christmas cooking." Visions of the world's largest turkey, plus enough trimmings to provide for all the families on the block, plus assorted goodies, which I could imagine after all these years of shopping with Tom, sent my adrenaline soaring!

"Let's go," I said quickly, hoping for the best. "I'm fine. I can make it.

The crowd was heavy, and we waited in line to walk down the aisles. I used the shopping cart as a giant crutch and leaned heavily as we selected the fruits and vegetables. Tom rushed off to bring small items, which I felt wouldn't cause him too much of a problem. The store was alive with all the Christmas shoppers, most of whom seemed to be my friends and neighbors. I stopped every few feet to chat.

"Hi, Liz! You look great. . . . How are you doing?"

"This is my first outing, and I'm getting tired," I responded. Then we would stand there and chat a bit before I continued down the aisles, choosing my fruits and vegetables between visits with my friends. Only halfway into our shopping, I surrendered the cart to Tom and went to wait for him in the car. I was sick with exhaustion and frustration, too, wondering how I was going to prepare this Christmas feast, when I could not stand long enough to gather in the food.

Thoughtfully, Tom had assembled all the ingredients for our customary batch of Christmas fudge; only this time it looked as though we would enjoy at least ten pounds of fudge!

"Really, dear, I don't think I can handle that big pan of candy," I told him, sadly. "We'll just have to forego the fudge this year."

"Nonsense," he replied, "I'll help you, and we'll get it done in no time. The children will be disappointed if you haven't made your great fudge." (. . . the children??) So it was that, at the age of fifty, Tom Munroe learned to make a batch of fudge; and he had such fun with the first, he made another! He was a marvelous help the following week with all the kitchen chores, from stuffing the turkey to scouring pots and pans. I love to cook, but I could certainly get used to having such a strong and capable assistant at my side as I do the creative stuff!

We made a list of chores, giving everyone a job, so the pace wouldn't get too hectic for the chef, who was still wobbly on her feet; each person was assigned a job for all the meals, including Christmas day, and even Aunty Dickie, who was joining us, would have an important task to perform in feeding our family of eight for the days we were together. One would scrub the potatoes, another could toss the salad, and Aunty was assigned to setting the table at every meal; then everyone would pitch in to help with the cleanup. As my mother was wont to say, "Many hands make light work," unfortunately just as all of us were tiptoeing out of the kitchen! Tom said that he wanted to volunteer for the dishwasher's job after the Christmas dinner, adding, "If the girls are unhappy with that, we'll just say that I am the only one who understands this kitchen!" I wanted to laugh, but he was so sincere that I didn't dare. We baked and cooked together, and we eventually reached the point when the refrigerator began to assume a very respectable appearance. We were ready for Christmas.

I was still resting several times a day, sometimes napping, other times content to sit on the loveseat by the bedroom window and enjoy the outdoor scene from that favorite sunlit nook. I watched the birds flutter into the unique ceramic feeder, which my friend, Gwen Redding, had made for me, and which Tom had hung from the limb of the tall sweet gum tree outside our bedroom window. One day I laughed at a tubby little squirrel who hung by his toes from the cord, swinging to and fro in his desperate attempt to reach the bird seed. I savored the beauty of the earth, happy with all God's creation. I enjoyed studying a white cyclamen plant sent to me by Sue White and her dear family, which lasted for months after it arrived, and I loved its crisp, dainty blossoms, each one like a little starched organdy bonnet. The plants seemed to burst their pots in great spurts of growth, and I felt the same spirit of stretching and reaching. Surely, I was more aware of all the goodness and beauty around me, more alive to the beautiful world God has created for us. I thought of the Lord often, with a fresh sense of gratitude.

"Hast thou not known? Hast thou not heard, that the everlasting God, the Lord, the creator of the ends of the earth, fainteth not, neither is weary? He giveth power to the faint; and to them that have no might he increaseth strength."

That is the strength I was experiencing every day.

CHAPTER NINE

"COMFORT YE, COMFORT YE MY PEOPLE, SAITH YOUR GOD. . . . PREPARE YE THE WAY OF THE LORD, MAKE STRAIGHT IN THE DESERT A HIGHWAY FOR OUR GOD.
. . . THE GLORY OF THE LORD SHALL BE REVEALED, AND ALL FLESH SHALL SEE IT TOGETHER:
HE SHALL FEED HIS FLOCK LIKE A SHEPHERD: HE SHALL GATHER THE LAMBS WITH HIS ARM, AND CARRY THEM IN HIS BOSOM, AND SHALL GENTLY LEAD THOSE THAT ARE WITH YOUNG."

Isaiah 40:1, 3b, 5a, 11

Laurie came home first. She was in high spirits, anticipating the holidays and the good food and rest she always enjoyed when the family was together.

"Mother!" she shrieked, before she even dropped her enormous bag of dirty clothes. "Is the Christmas tree still in the garage?" She was incredulous . . . three days before Christmas and the tree was still in the garage? "Can I put it up right now?"

I sank onto the couch, tiring at the sight of all that exuberance and energy.

"I'm sure Daddy will be glad to bring the ornaments from the garage, and I'm willing to help." I had been anxious to put the tree up myself, but it seemed an imposition on Tom with all he was doing already. He was not thinking now, surely, of taking boxes of decorations down from little-used corners of the garage, but it did have to be done. He was a good sport, and came in a few minutes with a huge box on one shoulder.

"I'll put the lights on for you, and after that you're on your own," he told Laurie. I was relegated to the couch, frustrated because decorating the Christmas tree was one of my favorite things, and I missed unwrapping the familiar ornaments which have been old faithfuls for many years.

The tree was the grandest and most beautiful we had ever had, so tall it touched the ceiling, so full it overflowed the corner where Tom placed it in the stand. We had a big tree this year because I became a tyrant for a brief moment! Tom is against big trees, and every year we tangle right there in the Christmas tree lot because I love a huge tree. This year, when Laurie came to visit one Saturday afternoon, she and Tom went to shop for our tree, with lots of instruction from me, taking advantage of my position in the bed.

"Please select a big tree . . . not one of those pines with the sharp needles . . . one of those gorgeous ones we admire when we camp in the Rockies . . . but get a BIG one," I commanded from the security of all my pillows. I was looking into Laurie's eyes, avoiding the flashing I knew was coming from Tom's.

"I deserve a big tree this year . . . blah, blah, blah"—I just couldn't quit. Oh, but what a tree they brought home! I couldn't have done better myself. It was the best tree we had ever had, and I was happy.

Now as Laurie unwrapped the shiny ornaments, exclaiming over each one as memories rushed back to her, I sensed her sadness at doing this task all alone. Obediently I lay on the couch, watching her and listening to her soft chatter, and I knew that she missed her brother and sister, who had always shared the fun of trimming the tree. Even her mother was incapacitated, and she felt alone.

When most of the bright balls had been hung with great care, a large pink one, a favorite, slipped from her hands and shattered at her feet. Instantly she burst into the most pitiful sobs, bringing Tom on the run from his study. He held her in his arms, soothing and speaking softly to her until her tears were spent. Later, as we talked together, we recognized that Laurie's burdens had been too heavy; her worries about me, as well as her final exams and her hospital work, had proven to be too much of a drain. At home, where she was secure and comfortable, she could allow herself the luxury of lowered defenses, and the tears had been a welcome release. We praised her Christmas tree enthusiastically and were uplifted in spirit by its beauty.

Christmas music is as much a part of our holiday tradition as stuffed turkey and mounds of fudge, with Handel's *Messiah* leading the other recordings as a favorite. I, especially, find that soaring, glorious music an inspiration, and, with the magnificent words taken directly from the Bible, it is an unchallenged combination:

> "Comfort ye, comfort ye my people, saith your God. . . . Prepare ye the way of the Lord, make straight in the desert a highway for our God. . . . And the glory of the Lord shall be revealed, and all flesh shall see it together. . . ."

And then that most lyrical and comforting of all music, music I am able to enjoy and thrill to over and over:

> "He shall feed his flock like a shepherd; he shall gather the lambs with his arm, and carry them in his bosom, and shall gently lead those that are with young."

Were there ever words more full of the meaning of a loving heavenly Father, of the feeling of gentle comfort and care? Once again, the music brought peace and joy into our hearts.

My bedtime schedule was still strange, and certainly out of kilter with a normal family routine; I found myself ready for bed about seven o'clock in the evening, and now was able to fall into the deepest sleep, waking in the early morning wondering where the night had gone. It was a happy change from the weeks I spent wandering about the darkened house in the night. When Aunty Dickie arrived from New York late one evening, I was already in bed, having disciplined myself to continue my schedule of proper sleep. Tom brought her home from the airport, along with her usual assortment of bags and bundles, packages for one and all, plus goodies like homemade yogurt and dried mint! When I greeted and hugged her, I sensed immediately her worry and concern about me. She was unable to conceal her distress at my condition, and, although she had come to help and comfort me, I found myself reassuring her in our days together. Watching as I exercised my arm using the rope over the door, she would turn away sadly, shaking her head in disbelief. When she felt I might be overdoing, preparing a meal, dusting, or sweeping, she became anxious and insisted that I go to bed.

"Aunty, I'm supposed to be using my arm so the muscles can get stronger and be reeducated," I told her often. "Please don't worry." Dr. L. had said that I should rest before I became tired and I found that to be valuable advice; however, she was not convinced.

Pris and Jack arrived next, followed closely by Chip and Karen, and now our family was complete. Our house was overflowing; I was delighted. Pris was surprised and encouraged to find me looking so well and behaving so normally.

"Mom, you look wonderful," she said, with feeling. "I'm so proud of you for the way you're handling this. Jack and I feel that this is our best Christmas ever!"

Her enthusiastic encouragement was heartwarming, and her matter-of-fact willingness to help wherever she was needed was the very boost her mother needed. Laurie relaxed visibly, too, obviously delighted to have big sister home, to relinquish some of the burdens she had borne alone. Karen had come bearing her homemade goodies, anxious to pitch in and help out, too. Tom and I shared the feeling that our cup was surely overflowing, and we thanked the Lord for our loving and faithful family.

So Christmas came for the Munroes, with its shining tree, the trays of good things to eat, with the stockings even hung by the chimney with care. It was fun and laughter, music and candlelight, but mostly it was love and hearts filled with gratitude. We rejoiced in our time together, thankful for the bonds which had pulled us back together. More than any other Christmas, I suppose, this one for me was heavy with the meaning of the coming of the Christ Child, and of the joy that is ours with the reception into our hearts of that Child. This Christmas was a month beyond my mastectomy, but I was strong in spirit, not because of my own puny efforts, but because, with Paul, I was able to say, "I can do all things through Christ which strengtheneth me." My body recovered in its own good time; however, throughout my physical recuperation, my spirit claimed that promise that He would be with us, even to the ends of the earth. My heart needed no more.

CONCLUSION

"BLESS THE LORD, O MY SOUL: AND ALL THAT IS WITHIN ME, BLESS HIS HOLY NAME. . . . WHO FORGIVETH ALL THINE INIQUITIES; WHO HEALETH ALL THY DISEASES . . . THE MERCY OF THE LORD IS FROM EVERLASTING TO EVERLASTING UPON THEM THAT FEAR HIM, AND HIS RIGHTEOUSNESS UNTO CHILDREN'S CHILDREN. . . . BLESS THE LORD, O MY SOUL."

Psalm 103

Sitting at the typewriter, this twentieth day of May, a fresh and sunny Sunday afternoon, I celebrate the six-month anniversary of my mastectomy. Many thoughts crowd my thinking. Primary, of course, is the fact of my recovery, physical as well as emotional, and the gratitude that is for me the natural response to that recovery. I have browsed the Psalms of praise and thanksgiving, hoping to borrow there the eloquence with which to express my own song of joy and thankfulness.

> "Make a joyful noise unto the Lord, all ye lands. Serve the Lord with gladness: come before his presence with singing . . . we are his people, and the sheep of his pasture. . . . Be thankful unto him, and bless his name. . . ."
>
> Psalm 100

> "O come let us sing unto the Lord; let us make a joyful noise to the rock of our salvation. Let us come before his presence with thanksgiving, and make a joyful noise unto him with psalms. . . . O come, let us worship and bow down: let us kneel before the Lord our maker. . . ."
>
> Psalm 95

> "Praise ye the Lord. Praise God in his sanctuary: praise him in the firmament of his power. Praise him for his mighty acts: praise him according to his excellent greatness . . . let every thing that hath breath praise the Lord. Praise ye the Lord."
>
> Psalm 150

> "I will extol thee, my God, O King; and I will bless thy name for ever and ever. Every day will I bless thee; and I will praise thy name for ever and ever . . . the Lord

upholdeth all that fall, and raiseth up all those that be bowed down. . . . The Lord is nigh unto all them that call upon him, to all that call upon him in truth . . . my mouth shall speak the praise of the Lord: and let all flesh bless his holy name for ever and ever."

Psalm 145

Each Psalm is more powerful and mighty than the one before; each one more beautiful in exultation and praise and thanksgiving than the next, and I cannot choose which one most nearly matches my own spirit of gratitude for the blessings that are mine in the Lord. I only know that, with the Psalmist, I will sing to the Lord as long as I live!

I remember that the 121st Psalm had been my father's favorite, and, whenever he spoke the words, eloquently, he stretched his arms heavenward, remembering the hills of his beloved Hadjin in the land of his birth:

> "I will lift up mine eyes unto the hills, from whence cometh my help. My help cometh from the Lord, which made heaven and earth. He will not suffer thy foot to be moved: he that keepeth thee will not slumber . . . the Lord is thy keeper: the Lord is thy shade upon thy right hand. The sun shall not smite thee by day, nor the moon by night. The Lord shall preserve thee from all evil. . . ."
>
> Psalm 121

". . . THY SHADE UPON THY RIGHT HAND . . . !" What a graphic description of the powerful and dynamic help for the people in a parched land! Even more exciting is the realization that the very same refuge preserves and protects those who trust in the Lord this day; those who have accepted that strength are still able to rely on that shade upon the right hand.

I have come through a season of trauma and pain, and, rejoicing now in my recovery, I continue life in gratitude to God for the present strength that is mine. I accept my body as it is, disfigured, yes, but functioning well again. I am excited about this book, remembering that the idea was not mine, and hoping that some may find comfort through it. Life continues and it is good. God has made us a wonderful world, there is much to be done in it, and there are many people who need our love;

there is so much for which to be grateful, and many songs to be sung. I sing from a grateful heart:

> "O give thanks unto the Lord, for he is good: for his mercy endureth for ever. Let the redeemed of the Lord say so. . . ."
>
> Psalm 107